Healing Your

# Ancestral

# Patterns

DAVID FURLONG

# HEALING YOUR ANCESTRAL PATTERNS

*How to access the past to heal the present*

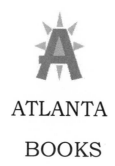

ATLANTA

BOOKS

**To my ancestors**

© 2014 David Furlong

First Published in 1997 as *Healing Your Family Patterns* by Judy Piatkus

This edition published in 2014

ISBN 978-0-9559795-4-5

Atlanta Books
Myrtles, Como Road,
Malvern, Worcestershire, WR14 2TH

www.atlanta-association.com

Ordering Information:
Special discounts are available on quantity purchases by corporations, associations, educators, and others. For details, contact the publisher at the above listed address.

A copy of the CIP entry for this book is available from the British Library

# Contents

# Acknowledgements

I wish to thank all those who have helped to formulate the ideas contained within this book and in particular the colleagues who have worked with me on the exploration of our ancestral patterns. In this context I particularly wish to thank April Taylor, Beatrice Duckworth, Karen Craig, Lady Mary Jardine, Shirley Newton, Jane Howell, Jan Morris, Joyce Harper, Paddy Clarke, Rosemary Atherton, Jackie Newton, Brian and Sheila Heaton-Ross and Gerri Kimber for their specific help and contributions. I also wish to thank my step-mother Nancy Furlong for her research in uncovering information on my own family tree. I would also like to thank Kathryn Logan and Semele Xerri for checking this current edition.

I acknowledge the valuable contributions of Deepak Copra, John Bradshaw, Monica McGoldrick, Randy Gerson, Rupert Sheldrake and Dr Motoyama to this field of research and for the extract from their works that I have drawn upon.

Finally I wish to express my gratitude to Dr Kenneth McAll, the author of *Healing Your Family Tree* for his insights as a pioneer in the field of ancestral healing and for the extracts from his book.

# *Foreword*

It is seventeen years since the publication of the first edition of *'Healing Your Family Patterns'*. During that time significant new developments have taken place in the field of genetics and the links that take us back to our ancient ancestral past. It has recently been discovered in a study that non-African humans have between 3-5% Neanderthal DNA in their genome. This stemmed from some inter-breeding between our ancestors and the Neanderthals after Homo-Sapiens left Africa around 70,000 years ago (Vermont and Akey, 2014).

Through studies in mitochondrial DNA we can now begin to plot the movement of peoples across the planet from that original exodus, so many thousand years ago. In his book the *Seven Daughters of Eve* Professor Bryan Sykes has shown that the bulk of the European population is descended from just seven women and that nearly half of the populace are the offspring of just one woman who lived in the South of France around 20,000 years ago (Sykes, 2001). Consider for a moment the sort of life she might have lived; the feelings she had; the challenges she faced? Although her life would have been outwardly different from what we experience today, inwardly she too would have had to face fears, deal with pain and loss and perhaps also enjoy the sunrise and the seasons, in a not too different way to how we experience the gamut of emotion that makes up our lives. Perhaps she is your clan mother? Certainly it would be someone similar if she were not, for you are descended from a long line of successful ancestors. Their trials and tribulations their successes and their failures are all woven into you as a seamless thread of experience.

We now know more about our early ancestors than ever before. The sequencing of the human genome in 2003 has lead to revolutionary new discoveries into the nature and origins of who and what we are. Additionally we now have access to online databases that allow us to begin to easily explore our direct ancestors and their descendants, where they lived, who they married and the children they bred. I recently tracked down a relative living in Stuttgart in Germany who was descended from a common ancestor who lived in 1800's. Television programmes like *'Who Do You Think You Are'* are enormously popular, for very many people are fascinated by their past. This may be because at an intuitive level they sense the importance of understanding their roots. New books such as *Healing Your Family History* (Hintze, 2006) and *The Ancestral Continuum* (O'Sullivan and Graydon, 2013) have provided further insights into the methods we can use to access into our rich heritage and also to clear patterns that are no longer appropriate for us.

Running alongside the studies of DNA has emerged a very new science called Epigenetics, which can be defined as the study of heritable changes that are **not** caused by changes in DNA sequence. It is now evident that the lives of our ancestors do leave clear imprints that are passed on down to us. This is an exciting new development because, when this book was originally written, it was not thought scientifically possible for behavioural patterns to be inherited. We now know that this is indeed what occurs and the mechanisms of this process are starting to be understood in the leading edge of genetic and epigenetic research (Spector, 2012). As this is a departure from the original text it was felt better to incorporate information on this enthralling field of study as a separate article in the Appendix at the end of the book under the theme of *'Epigenetics, Soul Essence and Ancestral Healing'*

This edition is a full update and revision on the previous edition incorporating the latest insights and findings and includes new exercises and case studies showing how you can link to your own family tree to clear the channels that flow down to you from your ancestors. It is now published under the original conceptual title, rather than the one chosen by the first publishers, as the theme relates more specifically to the ancestors rather than the immediate family. Additionally the contact list in the Appendix has been fully updated with current reference sources and organisations for support.

David Furlong
April 2014

# Introduction

We all have ancestors — real people who lived, breathed and experienced life, with similar emotions and feelings as ourselves. In some cases our forebears would have had happy, fulfilled lives; in others they would have died with feelings of guilt, anger, resentment, fear or remorse. You are the product of your ancestors, and something of the complex tapestry of their history is woven into you.

## Family patterns

Starting with your parents, your ancestral lineage doubles with each generation. Ten generations back and there are already over a thousand direct ancestors in your family tree. In a thousand years or thirty-two generations the number has reached a staggering 4¼ billion, over half the present world population. One generation more and it will have doubled again, so it is very easy to see that we are all ultimately related. Clearly any genetically based ancestral patterns will have their greatest impact in the first few generations.

Many people can remember one or even all of their grandparents, but very few meet their great-grandparents. Have you ever wondered what sort of characters yours might have been? They were probably born in the nineteenth century and would have lived a very different lifestyle from yours today. Yet despite the technological changes that have since taken place, the underlying themes of their lives would have been similar to those of your own. Human relationships, struggles to make ends meet and concerns over health were as relevant then as they are now. Whether your great-grandparents led contented, fruitful lives or were bowed down with the struggles of existence would have been dependent upon many factors, just as it is with you. Have you ever speculated on how much of their lives mirrors your own, or how much they might still be influencing you today?

In his book *Karma and Reincarnation* Dr Hiroshi Motoyama, head priest of the Shinto Tamamitsu sect of Japan, makes this profound statement:

> The parent/child connection manifests as one link in a long chain of ancestral karma that stretches back through time. Your link to your family allows you to be born into that specific line — it is a link that needs to be understood and respected. In this modern scientific age it is very difficult for people to accept the fact that they are responsible to their ancestors, that they are actually liable for the actions of their ancestors if the resulting karma has not yet been dissolved. Many find it absurd to think that the actions of an unknown ancestor could possibly have anything to do with what is happening to them today. But time and time again when investigating someone's karma, I find problems that stretch back generations. Their spirit is not just an individual entity, it is also part of the family spirit that births and nurtures it.

Science tells us that we inherit, through the genes, our physical shape, the colour of our eyes and hair, and to a lesser extent our mental and psychological make-up. Everything else, we are told, is the result of our life experiences. The nature/nurture debate (see Chapter 1) has been powerfully argued from both sides in academic circles since Darwin's time. In recent years family therapists have become aware of repeating patterns of behaviour and experience that appear to flow down through a number of generations, touching a member here and a member there. Clearly there is something deep at work in the dynamics of the family, which is now coming to light through the study of epigenetics.

Dr Motoyama suggests that occasionally we need to go back many generations to resolve family patterns, yet in practice it is the previous three generations, back to your great-grandparents, that are the most important. Including your parents, this makes fourteen individuals in all.

The central argument of this book, therefore, is that your immediate ancestors have passed on to you much more than physical attributes. The important facets of their lives, their successes, failures and temperaments, are also reflected in you. You are bound to them through powerful psychic forces, even if you know nothing of their lives.

Since her childhood, the author Murry Hope had been deeply fascinated by the Russian Revolution. Whenever she saw films or read stories about this period she found herself becoming agitated or very emotionally involved. At one point she thought that this might be a past-life memory, but many years later she discovered that one of her direct forebears had lived through the Revolution. At some level Murry felt that she was reliving or re-experiencing, through cellular memory, the feelings and perceptions of her deceased ancestor.

As we shall see in our exploration of this fascinating subject, the patterns of the past are no respecter of time.

The tapes of our ancestors' lives would appear to be replayed many times over during our own lifespan. This may seem a daunting or disturbing thought, but remember that these patterns do not always have to be detrimental: the positive qualities of our ancestors are also available to us.

## Healing through our forebears

This book will show not only the mechanisms of how the lives of our ancestors impact upon us, but also, more significantly, what can be done to change or heal dysfunctional patterns. Seeking to understand the causes of perceived psychological or emotional problems has encouraged therapists to look ever deeper into the innate patterns that we carry. Family therapists, in particular, have recognized the importance of ancestral dynamics as specific patterns from grandparents and great-grandparents weave down and across generations. In the many courses that I have run on the theme of ancestral healing I have never ceased to be amazed at the potency of energy that comes down to us from our ancestors, even in cases where individuals never knew their genetic parents or any of their family members.

My discovery of the need to address this aspect of human dynamics emerged from over twenty-eight years practice as a spiritual healer and counsellor. I had for a long time intuitively suspected that the psychological problems of some of my clients had ancestral origins. Despite this acknowledgement, I had never fully explored this aspect of healing until I came to write my book on healing which now goes under the title of *The Healer Within*. I realized that I could only legitimately introduce the subject of 'Ancestral Healing' into the book if I had carried out my own study. Fortunately at the time I was also running a number of training groups and together we set about the task of exploring our individual family patterns and what could be done to correct any dysfunctional elements.

To say that I was stunned by what emerged would be an understatement. It was like taking the lid off of a boiling cauldron that contained amazing potency. Clearly in my own case the steam from this pot had been seeping unconsciously into my life patterns since childhood. Removing the lid took away the pressure and allowed me the opportunity to sample and greatly improve the stew that had been brewing. So it was also for my colleagues and our resultant discoveries are now part of this book. Using the simple techniques given in this book, it is possible to ascertain which side of your family has the most powerful influence on your psyche and where imbalances lie.

In one particular case a client who suffered frequent irritating ailments had been aware for a long time of the possessive dominance of his father, which had caused him psychological problems. On the surface it was this that appeared to be the basis of his poor health. One session, using guided imagery and kinesthetic techniques, revealed that the origins of this problem lay not with the father but with the grandmother (his father's mother). Directing his attention to healing this ancestor produced a dramatic shift both in the client's relationship with his father and in his father's demeanour generally. This in turn led to a considerable improvement in the client's health. By healing his grandmother, he had in effect healed himself.

*To be truly whole we need to know ourselves, which means understanding all the factors that have been woven into our lives.*

Knowledge is power: by recognising ancestral patterns you have the opportunity of changing or transforming what is not appropriate. The exciting aspect of this transformative work is that you help not only yourself but all subsequent generations. But you cannot change what you do not perceive, so first you need to appreciate why your ancestors are important.

There is currently a strong movement to explore and understand the patterns that form our character. Many people are interested in the lives of their forebears —witness the large number of genealogical or family history societies and the courses that are run by local education authorities, as well as TV programmes such as *Who Do You Think Your Are?* For some this has become a fascinating pastime, involving considerable detective work in trying to trace back their family tree as far as they can. Other people may have an intuitive sense that their ancestral patterns are important without knowing quite why. In some situations a person might recognize a tendency to act in certain ways or to repeat particular patterns of behaviour when they discover that previous members of their family did the same thing. Other individuals have a strong sense that facets of their present inner conflicts might have arisen in previous generations.

In an article in the *Daily Mail* in February 1995 the well-known pop instrumentalist Mike Oldfield recounted how he had been working to uncover the origins of his psychological difficulties. He discovered that his grandfather had returned from the trenches in World War I a traumatized and radically changed man, and it was this that had laid the foundations for a great deal of suffering that ran down through the family. All the grandfather's four children had severe problems, and Oldfield's mother had sunk into an oblivion of alcohol, drugs and consequent electric shock treatment. To clear some of his own emotional problems he had to work with a therapist on resolving what his grandfather had set in motion.

In his book *Healing the Family Tree* Dr Kenneth McAll (1976), a consultant psychiatrist and an Associate Member of the Royal College of Psychiatrists, recounts the story of a woman who came to see him because she had developed a disturbing phobia about drowning. This had arisen after she saw her children tipping over in a boat, although they were only in a very shallow lake and in no danger. Research into her family tree revealed that an uncle of hers had drowned when the *Titanic* sank.

Dr McAll's method of treatment was, at an orthodox level, quite bizarre. He arranged for a memorial service to be held for the dead relative, in which his patient played an active part. When finished she felt completely free of her fear of drowning. By healing an ancestor she had effectively healed herself. Interestingly, in this case it was not even a direct forebear, yet the story beautifully captures the spirit of family responsibility that Dr Motoyama suggests we carry. It offers hope for healing those impediments that come down to us through the family tree. This book is dedicated to that process and offers the exciting prospect that when we heal the past we also heal the future. In other words releasing family karma, or family patterns, not only clears the situation for yourself but also releases its hold on future generations.

## Ancestral Patterns of Nation States

As well as individual family karma, we are also connected both into the ancestral karma of the country in which we reside as well as the ethnicity from which we have emerged. These patterns can be evidenced most powerfully within some cultures such as the Jewish but also touch all of us from time to time. Great national traumas such as the Irish Potato famine can leave an indelible mark on the psyche of the people and these get passed on to future generations. Since the first publication of this book some groups have taken on the task of sending healing to some of these group family/country traumas, which affected thousands of individuals. Within Britain and Europe, over the past century, there has been the devastation of two world wars, which has left a deep scar. Sadly these types of situations are still being created or worked out at present, as evidenced by what is happening in Syria and in some Islamic countries, like Iraq. Rivalries between the Sunnis and the Shias, which had its origins in ancestral conflicts, still give rise to bloodshed today.

## The value of ancestral healing

There are, then, three predominant reasons why you will benefit considerably from spending time accessing and healing your ancestral patterns. It will help you:

- Gain insight into yourself and the innate patterns that are part of your life
- Resolve any family karma, freeing up conditions for future generations
- Heal specific illnesses or conditions that stem from your forebears

This may seem a challenging task, particularly if you are already working on difficult childhood issues or past life conditions. But in practice it need not be too onerous. Indeed, there is a powerful dynamic that comes to the fore when you work on helping others, and by diverting attention from yourself to past members of your family you will often resolve previously blocked situations. In my experience many parent/child problems have their origins in ancestral patterns. The answer to changing some of the dynamics of your life might only be found through working on your family tree.

With some people dramatic changes occur — such as the removal of the phobia of drowning mentioned previously — particularly when dealing with emotional or psychological issues. In others the shifts are much less obvious, although still important, as new insights and perceptions become woven into their lives. In the many courses on this theme that I have run, and in work with my private clients, I have never met an individual who has not felt enriched by the experience of connecting into their ancestral heritage.

## The scientific perspective

Ancestral patterning can be seen in two ways:

- We carry within our genetic structure the make-up of our ancestors, which includes emotional and psychological tendencies as well as our physical structure
- A psychic bond exists, which bridges across time, linking family members together

Each of these ideas will be examined in greater depth during the course of this book. These two concepts stand at the very frontier of present scientific knowledge, or even beyond it, so one of the tasks here will be to present sufficient evidence to show how these ideas might be contributing to the patterns that shape your life.

The current consensus of science is that all hereditary traits stem from the DNA molecule. Genetic research stands at the leading edge of biological studies, and discoveries are regularly made that herald the hope of finding a cure for some hereditary diseases. Mapping our DNA is now big business, with vast sums of money being spent to discover its potential benefits. However, ancestral patterning suggests that a different model may be required — that instead of being repositories of encoded information, the genes themselves may only rebroadcast what originates from another source, level or field (just as a radio is not the source of the information that it broadcasts). This idea, postulated by Rupert Sheldrake in his theories of morphogenetic fields, will be explored more fully in Chapter 4. Since the turn of the millennium, new studies into the field of epigenetics have provided more insights into how the DNA works within us, showing how we can adapt the patterning of our genome. These exciting new discoveries, which only emerged after *Healing Your Family Patterns* was published, will be fully covered in the Appendix.

## Working with this book

Part 1 of this book looks at the different beliefs that surround our ancestors as well as exploring the role of DNA in our genetic make-up and the ways of drawing up family trees. There is also much evidence from family therapy on the patterns of experience or dysfunction that weave down, through and across generations. Chapters 1-5 aim to pull together some of these many threads of belief and insight from the various therapeutic, scientific and spiritual disciplines.

In Part 2, the focus is on the different methods that you can adopt to change any undesirable inherited influences. You may wonder what these might be, or you may already be aware of some of your hereditary patterns. A little time and effort in this direction can be very rewarding, even if you feel healthy and well balanced yourself. I have been amazed at what has come up, even within well-adjusted people, and at the valuable opportunities that have emerged for healing some past problem.

I am suggesting two things here:

- If some kind of disease or disharmony is making itself felt upon your life, whether it be physical, emotional, mental or spiritual, its origins may be ancestral. This is particularly so if other members of your family carry or experience similar traits.
- Secondly, from a larger perspective we all carry a level of responsibility for our family karma. If the greatest benefit is to flow into ourselves as well as into our children or other family members, healing the family tree is an important part of the process because it frees up energies for both present and future generations. How much better to incarnate into a family that holds only positive karma! If those who espouse the concept of reincarnation are correct, that soul may be you.

Finally this book approaches the themes of ancestral healing from a spiritual perspective. In other words a key component is not just the patterns of experience that stem from your forebears but your inherent personality that stems from what might be called your soul essence. As we shall see, even with identical twins, which have the same DNA, there is still a strong sense of individuality and uniqueness that makes each twin distinctly different. It is argued here that this difference stems from your inner spiritual and eternal self. It is by learning to access this part of our being that we can directly influence and shape the manifestation of our family patterns.

# PART 1

## *Mapping the Territory*

## CHAPTER 1

# The Role of Our Ancestors

To make sense of why our ancestors are important in our own lives we must briefly examine the nature of who and what we are. For generations, scientists have debated the nature versus nurture issue — heredity or environment. Both are important factors, but which of the two is more dominant has taxed the minds of many thinkers. Opinion over the years has shifted regularly from one pole to the other, depending on current research and the climate of political belief. In Nazi Germany, for instance, genetics was the prime factor, which led to belief in Aryan supremacy and the inferiority of other races. In socialist regimes, on the other hand, environment and upbringing are seen as the main shapers of culture. On an individual level this can be summarized into trying to determine how much the pattern or outcome of your life is the result of the environmental influences of your upbringing and how much is the result of your genetic inheritance.

## The missing factor

Yet within this fascinating debate one central point is always ignored: the influence of your spiritual self or life essence, the motivating facet that resides in all living things. At its simplest level it is what determines whether an organism is alive or dead. Within human beings it has been given a number of names, but whether you choose to call it your higher consciousness, soul or some other term is of no matter. Its importance lies in the way in which it injects a crucial third dimension into the nature/nurture equation.

The question that then arises is how this element affects or modifies the other two aspects. To attempt any meaningful assessment, we need to examine the evidence from those who have stood at the threshold of death and had what has become known as a near death experience or NDE.

## Near Death Experience

Many people are now familiar with this concept — an experience that almost always has a profound effect on those involved. The person in question is consciously aware of being detached from his or her body and seeing their surroundings from a very different level of perception. For example they might view their physical self from above, witnessing the efforts of medical staff trying to revive them. Sometimes they will also undergo an apparent transfer to another plane of reality where they experiences feelings of great peace and sometimes meet deceased relatives or other individuals, who communicate with them. At this point they might be informed that it is not yet time to die, and they then find themselves being drawn back into their body.

Here is a typical example taken from a *Daily Mail* article in 1995 by Graham Turner. It recounts the experiences of a woman in her mid-forties who very nearly died from pneumonia. Passing from her body, she travelled down a tunnel of light and then found herself standing in a beautiful field. The story continues:

> *On my right was a wooden bench, the sort that you see around playing fields. It hadn't got any arms on it. There sat my Grandpa Tuck who died eight years before. I went over and sat next to him.*
>
> *`Are you all right, girl?' he asked.*
>
> *`Yes,' I replied, 'I'm fine.' He was as real to me as my daughter Angela. He was dressed as he used to be, old*

*cloth cap, jacket and working overalls, as if he hadn't died at all. It's really weird looking back on it.*

*I told him I didn't want to go back. 'You've got to go, girl,' he said, 'for the sake of the kids.' I couldn't bear the thought and I wasn't worried about the kids either. I remember thinking that my husband was quite capable. I said: 'You will come back for me when my time comes, won't you?' and he said: 'Yes, I'll be back after four ... ' Then there was a kind of electric shock, and I came back in intensive care.*

This story suggests that the grandfather was well aware of what was happening to both his granddaughter as well as her children, and had a sense of what was best for their future.

In almost every case the person who returns from a NDE loses all fear of death, and has a strong sense of the continuity of his or her existence. From this moment death is perceived as a wonderful transition into another state of existence. These experiences support the idea that part of our consciousness survives the death of the physical body and continues to exist in some other dimension. If we continue to exist after death, did we also exist before birth?

## Do we return again?

A number of religious beliefs suggest that some souls, at least, return into a new body or reincarnate. Perhaps the most authoritative researcher in this field is Professor Ian Stevenson of the University of Virginia, who has conducted exhaustive enquiries into claims of memories from previous lives. Whilst maintaining an open mind on this subject, he has concluded that it is very difficult to explain some cases other than by asserting that part of our inner consciousness can inhabit or return to another body. In some of these cases he has witnessed birthmarks, or physical defects, which exactly match the fatal injuries suffered by that person in their remembered previous life. In one particular case an Indian child who was able to describe accurately many facets of his previous life, even visiting his former home, had in his former existence died from a bullet wound in his temple. In his present life a birthmark on his temple indicated the exact position of the original fatal wound (Stevenson, 1974).

This suggests that your inner consciousness can influence the structural make-up of your body. Since the latter is created by your DNA, it can therefore change or modify your genetic inheritance or at least the way that it expresses itself. This is an intriguing prospect.

Clearly the extent of these changes is limited, for offspring do not display totally different traits from their parents. Yet if this reincarnation theory is correct it might explain some of the differences in temperament that arise between identical twins. For, in theory at least, identical twins brought up in the same household should display very similar character traits, yet in practice they often have very different temperaments. However, as we shall see in Chapter 4, twin studies also throw up some other fascinating anomalies.

## The dynamics of life

Following this line of thinking, I suggest that there are three primary forces or patterns that operate through your life. These are:

- the patterning that comes from your environment, which includes your upbringing
- the patterning that comes through your genetic make-up, which includes all ancestral influences
- the patterns that stem from your inner consciousness or spiritual self, which includes past-life and personal karmic patterns

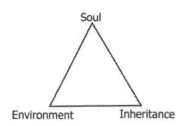

Soul

Environment    Inheritance

Each of these three elements has an important part to play in determining the direction of your life, and each needs to be seen as an integral part of the equation that makes you who and what you are. Any or all of these three might be contributory factors in ill health.

# Do our ancestors still exist?

If your consciousness survives the death of the physical body, as many religions attest and the NDE evidence supports, then your ancestors must continue to exist on some plane of existence or perhaps they have already reincarnated. But do they still have some influence upon us, and if so in what way? There could be a direct feeling of intervention, as in the case of healing energy being channelled by the ancestors to their kin (see p. 18). Or there may just be a caring overview as suggested by the grandfather in the NDE case. If the ancestors' consciousness, on whatever plane they exist, is locked into an inner trauma, more destructive influences may be generated. Some ancestral imprints may therefore be benign, whilst others may not be so beneficial. This principle correlates closely with many worldwide beliefs on the way the ancestors impact upon our lives.

### Spiritualism

Direct communication between the spirit world and the earthly plane is one of the main features of Spiritualist belief. Founded in 1848 in America, the movement swept through both the USA and Britain and reached its height at the end of the nineteenth century when it boasted some 2 million adherents. At Spiritualist meetings mediums in different stages of trance connect to the souls of the 'loved ones' and relay messages to specific individuals in the audience. In the majority of cases these messages are aimed at proving the existence of the soul after death, so they generally come from close relatives who have recently 'passed over'.

The millions of communications that have been delivered over the years can act only as anecdotal information that is very hard to verify or deny. Certainly these messages generally give comfort to those looking for a belief in an afterlife. It is also clear that the ancestors are mostly concerned with the day-to-day lives of their relatives. The most frequent type of communication does not involve the ancestors' life in the celestial realm, or even the spiritual life of the living relatives, but more pragmatically what they should be doing practically in their daily life. The type of clothes to wear, the food to eat, dangers to watch out for and so on are the main thrust of the ancestors' relayed advice. Interestingly this idea also accords, in essence, with the more ancient tradition of ancestor worship, which generally espouses the notion that the ancestors' primary concern is the physical wellbeing of their living relatives.

## Ancestor worship and native wisdom

Although ancestor worship is incorporated even today into both primitive societies and more sophisticated ones such as the Chinese, in Western culture it is not generally an accepted practice. This is perhaps the result of Christian attempts down the centuries to overturn established pagan beliefs.

Those cultures which revere and worship their ancestors, however, believe that they can still play a valuable part in assisting the wellbeing of the living relatives. In societies and times where life was hard it was wise to seek as much support as possible — if it made good psychological sense. Yet we should not dismiss these beliefs out of hand. Native peoples show an awareness of other realms of existence that are not obvious to their more educated observers. The explorer Laurens Van Der Post, for example, found that the bushmen of the Kalahari Desert in Southern Africa knew in advance which of several pilots would be flying the aircraft that used their landing strip, even though there was no direct radio communication. The villagers were aware also, through some form of telepathic communication, when one of their hunters had killed an eland, a very special event, and immediately set in motion preparations for a celebratory feast (Van Der Post, 1958). Similar abilities have been recounted by anthropologists in different parts of the world, particularly amongst the Aborigines of Australia and Native Americans. Even individuals in Western societies have seen ghosts or experienced similar types of psychic phenomena — so these native peoples, whose telepathic sense is much greater, must have had considerable experience of them.

In my own life I have witnessed many forms of channelled communication with deceased people. I have also had my own direct experiences where information has been given, and later verified, that I did not know at the time. On the first visit that my ex-wife Diane made to a medium that she had never met or communicated with previously, she was told that her recently deceased Uncle Jim was present. He wanted Diane to pass on a message to her father, Jim's brother, that he was OK. The accuracy of the description, his name and other details tallied exactly with the uncle whom Diane knew, and who had only died a few months earlier. It was impossible for this information to have been known to the medium prior to Diane's visit. It was either an extraordinary guess, or an accurate description of what this ancestor was wishing to convey.

Although we are members of a technologically advanced society, we should not thoughtlessly dismiss what 'native wisdom' might have to tell us. Today, scientists are beginning to re-examine what was previously dismissed as superstitious nonsense. Orthodox medicine now has to compete with a vast array of complementary therapies that include acupuncture, homeopathy, reflexology, radionics, crystal therapy and spiritual healing. All these systems lie outside the range of orthodox scientific understanding. According to current scientific theory they should not work, but the weight of empirical evidence suggests that they do. It is my contention that native peoples' insight into the role of our ancestors has something important to teach us.

## Ancestral help in healing

Within many cultures the ancestors were seen as an integral part of the healing process. They were invoked when specific help was required and propitiated when their influences were felt to be less than benign. A modern doctor watching a native healing ceremony, which requested the ancestors' intervention could be forgiven for wondering if any beneficial results might only be suggestion — the placebo effect. Indeed this must be part of the process, for all beliefs have their impact. But the shaman or witch doctor carrying out the ceremony would claim that the ghosts or souls of the ancestral spirits were actually participating in the event. Their energy, their presence, would be sensed in a very real, powerful and dramatic way.

The author and researcher, Peter Dawkins, who happens to be very psychic, witnessed such a ceremony amongst the Xavante Indians of the Matto Grosso in Brazil. The chief of this tribe had been forewarned in a dream that Peter and his friends would be visiting the village and that they were to be made welcome. When the party arrived they were told that a special healing ceremony was to be enacted that evening for a young girl who had been sick for a month. The chief informed the gathering that the ceremony would last all night and at daybreak the child would be well. A fire was lit and the warriors lined up in a semi-circle on one side with the child on the other. They then started to dance, chanting a particular song to their ancestors.

After a short while the girl was led back into a hut and Peter's group took her place in the circle. He started to watch, through his inner psychic vision, what was taking place. The rhythm of the dance and song created an energy that acted as a bridge between this world and the next. Peter was aware that an inner connection was being made through the ancestors, to a higher or finer level of healing energy. Eventually he became aware of a great 'being of light' handing down a powerful healing energy, through the ancestors, to those participating in the ceremony. Just before dawn the child was brought forward again and this time Peter 'saw' the vision of what he took to be the child's grandmother gather this energy together and present it to the child, whereupon she immediately got up and appeared free of her ailment. At that point the shaman and the chief gave thanks for the help they had received.

Reflecting on this experience, Peter questioned the necessity of all the ritual and preparation and in particular the connection with the ancestors in this ceremony. 'Would it not be easier to make direct contact to the "being of light"?' he mused. A few weeks later, back in England, he was struck down by a malaria-type illness. A healer friend suggested that he imagine himself back in Brazil, as the child in the ceremony. He did so, and immediately felt a healing energy enter his body and take away the symptoms.

An echo of his previous question came into his mind. 'Why were the ancestors necessary?' The 'being of light' appeared to respond by saying that, whilst it is possible to connect to the source of healing without ancestral support, invoking the ancestors allowed them to assist in an experience which benefited everyone. In this way it became a much more holistic process. At that moment Peter became aware of his mother, who had died about six months previously, standing by his side. She was overjoyed at the opportunity to participate. Coincidentally, as it later transpired, the chief of the Xavante 'knew' that Peter and one or two of his friends were ill, and had organized another healing ceremony, by proxy, for them. Such experiences cannot be lightly dismissed.

## Genetic healing

In orthodox science ancestral powers are perceived only through the workings of the DNA molecule and our hereditary make-up. Until quite recently the consensus was that, once the genetic code was established at the moment of conception, it stayed immutably fixed throughout our life unless altered through radiation or genetic engineering. Effectively we could not change what nature had endowed us with — only make the best of what we had been given. But now this position cannot be so rigidly defended, for there are anomalies which suggest that the genetic code can be modified or at least that its messages can be changed.

In the mid-fifties a young boy with a severe skin problem was diagnosed as having a serious outbreak of warts. His doctor heard that hypnotism sometimes worked in these cases and referred him to Dr Mason, a clinical hypnotist at the Queen Victoria Hospital in East Grinstead. The boy proved to be an excellent subject, and through hypnotic suggestion his condition began to clear up. In the meantime, just to be sure that the original diagnosis was correct, a sample of skin tissue was analysed. The results revealed that the boy was suffering not from warts, which are caused by a virus, but from congenital ichthyosis or fishskin disease, a hereditary condition for which there was no known cure (Mason, 1956).

In theory it was impossible for the boy to have made any recovery just through the suggestions of the hypnotist; yet the results were there for all to see. Certainly the hypnotist thought at first that he was dealing with warts and therefore believed strongly in the possibility of a cure. Over the next four years a 60-70 per cent permanent improvement was achieved. This would suggest that it is possible, under the right circumstances, for the messages coming from our genetic code to be modified by our thought processes.

One sophisticated culture that has provided a coherent link between the role of the ancestors and healing is that of the Chinese. Their many therapeutic systems, such as acupuncture and shiatsu, give insight into how ancestral patterns might reveal themselves within us.

## Chinese medicine and the ancestors

In Chinese medicine, all illness is said to be caused by imbalances between two principles that, as well as existing within us, are found in all things. These are known as yin and yang and are portrayed graphically by a solid line — (yang) and a dashed line – – (yin). Yang contains all that is outward, strong, active, masculine and expansive. It is the positive pole on an electrical circuit. Conversely yin holds all that is receptive, yielding, passive, feminine and inward. It is the negative pole on the electrical circuit. Through acupuncture, herbs, diet or some other remedy a Chinese physician would endeavour to balance these two dynamic energies within his patient. These yin/yang principles are considered to express themselves through three primary forces known as Ch'i, Shen and Jing.

The yin/yang symbol

The energy of Ch'i, according to the Chinese, is one of the main sources of vitality for the body and is predominantly held within the environment. We draw Ch'i into ourselves through food, in the air we breathe, in liquids and through other subtle environmental influences. Shen is the energy of your spirit or soul and gives power and flavour to your life. Jing relates to sexual energy but also holds the stored power from your ancestors. For good health all these energies need to be in balance, and it is the task of the traditional Chinese doctor continually to monitor these three forces. This is a very interesting concept for, as previously mentioned, it incorporates the notion of a triangle of energies — spirit, environment and genetics — that weave through all facets of your life. We should not forget that the Chinese systems of healing were initiated nearly four thousand years ago; so it would appear, in some aspects at least, that they could well be ahead of us in their thinking.

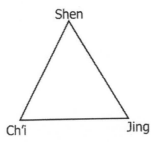

As well as the innate patterns of Jing, the Chinese are aware of their ancestral spirits, and spend much time revering and communicating with them. These spirits are perceived as real presences that connect to the family, acting as its guardians or supporters. As in the West, disturbed spirits or ghosts sometimes cause the family problems, and at such times special help is sought from a doctor or shaman.

In traditional Chinese belief, then, the ancestral patterns have two aspects. One is the ancestral energy (Jing) which flows through the individual, and which we could equate loosely with our genetic make-up; the other is the spiritual presence of that ancestor and its impact on both the family and the individual. It is this latter aspect that is most widespread throughout different cultures, and a whole range of beliefs were orientated towards acknowledging, appeasing or invoking specific ancestors for help. This idea will be looked at more closely in Chapter 2, but it is worth mentioning here that some cultures perceived all ancestral influences as the forces of destiny created by specific acts of the ancestors whilst they were alive. These patterns were seen as family karma that flowed down through the generations. Judaic belief and therefore some elements of Christianity too, fall into this category.

## Ancestral links in the Judaeo-Christian ethic

In the Bible we read that 'the sins of the fathers will be visited upon the children even unto the third and fourth generation'. (Exodus 20:5). In the New Testament the disciples asked Jesus of the man born blind, 'Who did sin? This man or his parents that he was born blind?' In this case Jesus was quite unequivocal when he stated: `Neither hath this man sinned nor his parents: but that the works of God should be made manifest in him.' (John 9:1-3). This statement is often quoted by those who believe in reincarnation as evidence that Christ and the disciples accepted the concept of pre-existence, as well as the notion that the misdeeds of the parents could be inflicted upon future generations — the argument being that the disciples would never have posed such a question if they had not themselves firmly believed that the origins of the condition must lie either with the sins of the father or from some sin (karma) from pre-birth, which by implication suggests a past life. In this particular case Christ offers an alternative explanation yet without refuting the original concept.

In another story the prophet Elisha curses his servant Gehazi for having deceitfully obtained money from Naaman, whom Elisha had just healed of leprosy, with the words: '*The leprosy of Naaman shall cleave unto thee, and unto thy seed forever.' And he went out from his presence a leper as white as snow.* (2 Kings 5:27). This supports the idea of the misdeeds of an ancestor running down through generations, in this case causing disease.

In some cases dysfunctional patterns would appear to stalk through many generations. Perhaps the most powerful example is the enmity between the Jews and the Arabs. Both trace their descent back to Abraham. In the biblical story we are told that God promised Abraham that he would be a father of many nations and that his wife Sarah would give birth to a son. Because she was so old Sarah did not believe that she could conceive and had given to Abraham, as a mate, her maid-servant Hagaar. A son called Ishmael was eventually born to Hagaar. When Ishmael was thirteen years old God reaffirmed his promise to Abraham, and the next year Sarah bore a son who was called Isaac. Ishmael would now have been fourteen — a number that has some significance, as will be seen later. Unfortunately Hagaar and Sarah quarrelled, and so Hagaar was cast out and nearly died with her son. But she too was protected by God and survived. Today the Jews trace their descent through Isaac, whilst the Arabs believe they are descended from Ishmael. It is interesting to speculate on the family karma that has come down through so many generations, holding these two great peoples in such strife.

## Tribes, clans and races

Our allegiance to our clan, tribe or race can be very powerful, and the energies generated will sometimes propel individuals into acts of aggression that on a rational level are quite out of proportion. Aside from the Arab—Israeli enmity just mentioned, many other present wars on the planet have tribal overtones: the conflicts in Bosnia, Northern Ireland and Ruanda are all rooted in ancient ethnic or religious differences.

It is quite feasible that collective ancestral energy is the motivating force that drives people to act in this way. Blood relationships would appear to have powerful bonding qualities that perhaps originated when there was a need to protect the group from invaders. In a similar context, the incidence of child abuse is highest when either the father or mother is a step-parent for it is thought that powerful biological forces invoke strong protective feelings for one's own genetic offspring, which are absent between step-parent and child. Letting go of destructive tribal loyalties could be regarded as an aspect of ancestral healing.

## Healing family patterns

There are three distinct facets to healing ancestral patterns:

- The role of the ancestors themselves: the sort of lives that they led, and what influences they might be exerting from beyond the grave. If these are not beneficial, what can be done to ameliorate or change their impact
- Your own unique genetic make-up as encoded in your DNA, and what methods might be adopted to modify any conflicting patterns
- The facet that Dr Hiroshi Motoyama has called family karma, which can perhaps best be seen as a form of psychic family link. These links may need resolution or severing so that the karma is broken

The methods explained in this book will address each of these specific areas.

Two further ideas might be considered helpful. The first is the way in which we regard our ancestral spirits. Rather than just seeing them as disembodied souls, moving between the spiritual world and this earth, we could consider them as patterns or fields of energy that contain all the experiences of the original ancestor. It might not then be the ancestor that affects us but the patterns of energy that they left behind. This idea may strike a chord with people who have problems with the concept of family ghosts wandering around their home.

The second and perhaps more fundamental point is that all patterns can be altered. Just because an event from the past set in motion a particular pattern it does not necessarily mean to say that it is fixed and immutable. In the same way that a scientist can modify patterns through changing the genetic structure, a great deal can be done to rectify ancestral patterns. By healing the influences that come down to us from our ancestors we can change the way that we act and react to situations. Instead of being helpless in the face of these dynamic forces, we can do some influencing back, so that impaired past patterns are corrected, cycles broken and the future improved.

## CHAPTER 2

# *The Ancestors in Religion and Myth*

To appreciate what role your own ancestors may be playing in your life we need to explore in more detail how they are perceived in other cultures.

This chapter looks at some of the worldwide beliefs and myths that involve ancestor worship in one form or another. It is a widespread phenomenon, with many cultures recognizing some kind of ancestral impact upon their lives. Ancestor worship is found extensively among simple societies but is also an integral part of Taoism, Confucianism, Shintoism and some of the Eastern Buddhist sects. The ancestors are usually of two kinds: tribal heroes and family ancestors.

Tribal ancestral spirits embody the great heroes or founding fathers of the tribe. These are the beings who protect the whole clan or group and are worshipped as such. In one sense they could be perceived in the same way that a Christian would worship Christ or a Buddhist reveres the Buddha. Often these ancestral spirits are endowed with magical powers, which can be called upon for healing, protection or fertility.

Family ancestral spirits include, deceased parents, uncles and aunts, grandparents and great-grandparents who might still have an interest in the lives of their living family. The ancestors' great advantage over incarnate relatives is their access to the spirit world and to higher spirit beings. In this role they can act as valuable intermediaries when special help is required. They can also protect their living relatives from evil spirits, which amongst superstitious people are always a hazard.

From a scientific standpoint it is fair to argue that these different belief systems might have arisen because of an intuitive awareness of genetic patterning that could not be explained in any other way except through some form of 'ancestral spirit' involvement. Without knowledge of genetics, the tendencies of children to behave in similar ways to their forebears could only be understood in terms of the ancestors influencing descendants.

## Tribal ancestors

The Cherokee tribe from North America believe they are descended from a race of beings called the Nunnehi, who were described as gourd-headed, hairless and tall. These beings could move through the natural elements at will. The Cherokee have many stories of men becoming enamoured of a disguised Nunnehi and then attempting to follow her home, only to be bewildered when she disappeared into a rock or lake. These Nunnehi do what they can to protect the tribe in a benevolent way, and certain places are held sacred as their homes.

The Nunnehi seem to possess many similar qualities as the Kachinas of the Hopi people, also from North America. The Hopi Kachina ceremonies involve some of the most famous of all the Native American dances. They are woven around secret night-time rituals held in their underground sanctuaries known as Kivas, before the Hopi emerge at dawn to dance to their gods. The Kachinas are worshipped as star beings, who originally came from the constellation known as the Pleiades. They have assumed many different guises which are depicted in Kachina dolls. In their beliefs and myths, the Hopi affirm that they are guided by the Kachinas in all aspects of their lives. Today the Kachinas are believed to reside in the San Francisco Peaks in Arizona, and many ceremonies to invoke their help are held every year.

The Gilbert Islanders from the Pacific distinguish two types of beings whom they propitiate. They are the gods *(anti)* and the divine ancestors *(anti-ma aomata)*. Living people *(aomata)* have to perform rituals to both groups, but are most anxious to appease the divine ancestors. One of the original ancestors who was especially invoked was Taburimai, the first human offspring of the fish gods. He sailed around the islands, took a wife and brought civilization to the people. His son, Te-ariki-ntarawa, climbed the sacred tree of heaven and married the tree goddess. It was claimed that all mankind descended from these two ancestors.

## The divine ancestor as king

In some cases the king embodied an aspect of the divine ancestor. In Ancient Egypt the Pharaoh was seen as the incarnation of the falcon-headed god Horus, son of Isis and Osiris, who battled with the evil god Set for his father's throne. Likewise in Peru the king or Inca was perceived as the incarnation of the sun god Inti, the supreme deity. The Shang kings who founded the state of China around 1650 BC were regarded as the sons of heaven, ruling on behalf of Shang Di, the supreme celestial god. Only they possessed the authority to beg the ancestral spirits for blessings. The concept of the divinity of kings has an echo in the notion of the 'divine right', believed in by certain British monarchs, which conferred on them the ability to heal the disease scrofula, also known as the King's Evil.

## Destructive ancestors

Not all tribal ancestors brought benefit to the world. The Ngombe tribe of Africa believed that Akongo, the supreme god of the sky, put the goddess Mbokomo into a basket and lowered her to the earth with her son and daughter. The family planted a garden, which flourished. The mother then persuaded the son to sleep with the daughter to procreate children, which they did. But the daughter also slept with a creature called Ebonga, who practised magic and witchcraft, and it was their child which brought evil into the world. This myth has an echo in the biblical story of Adam and Eve and suggests that somewhere within the human psyche is the notion that evil originated from some misdeed in the past, although different cultures give divergent accounts of what this might be.

In a Hawaiian myth, the divine ancestress of the people was called Papa, which means flat. She was associated with the underwater foundations of the Hawaiian islands and was the supreme earth goddess. Papa married Wakea, the first chieftain, and bore him many children, whom she showered with her blessings. Sadly, Wakea indulged in an incestuous relationship with one of his daughters; as a result Papa left the earth in rage and cursed mankind with death.

### Ghost dances

In times of crisis the people would call upon their tribal ancestors to protect them. The power of this belief was demonstrated in the famous 'ghost' dance ceremonies of the Native American, which arose in response to the relentless onslaught of the whites. The cult started in 1888 when a Paviotso Indian called Wovoka had visions which gave rise to a doctrine that contained Christian ethics as well as a strong belief in the disappearance of the white man, the return of the buffalo that the white man had virtually wiped out, and the resurrection of dead tribal members. Wovoka specifically preached nonviolence. News of his visions reached the Plains tribes, many of whom were at this time on the verge of starvation. They took up part of Wovoka's message but saw their only solution to be war against the whites. By dancing in a circle and calling upon their ancestors they believed that they would become immortal: that the power of the rituals alone would be sufficient to ward off bullets and bring back the buffalo. Some of the Sioux, the Arapaho, Cheyenne and Kiowa adopted the doctrine completely. It was a situation that could not last, and it ended with the final defeat of the Plains Indians at the infamous Battle of Wounded Knee.

## Heroes, saints and lesser gods

In Egyptian, Greek and Roman mythology, heroes were sometimes elevated to the status of minor gods. In Egypt only two individuals were accorded this accolade: Imhotep, who was responsible for the building of the step pyramid of King Zoser, and the xiv dynasty sage and philosopher Amenhotep son of Habu. Some authorities have suggested that it was Amenhotep, who inspired the religious and artistic reforms of the Pharaoh Akhenaten. Greek heroes such as Orion, Perseus and Hercules had their effigies placed in the stars for all to see and worship.

As time developed great ancestors became acknowledged as part of humanity and were no longer restricted to any particular local tribe. Some of these ancestors led lives or displayed some talent that has acted as inspiration to thousands of people across many cultures. Many religious groups, including Buddhists, Christians and Moslems, have their 'saints' who are called upon to intercede on behalf of the supplicant. Their homes or the sites of the visionary visitation, such as Lourdes, have become centres of worship and healing.

## Family ancestors

These ancestors are generally taken to mean relatives have died relatively recently. Within many cultures it was the family ancestors who were the most important, requiring full acknowledgement and correct propitiation. It was they who could bring the greatest benefit or detriment to the family.

Although they were perceived as existing in the spirit, they would act in a very similar way to when they were alive: the deceitful ancestor did not suddenly become truthful just because he or she had died. It was therefore important to know the qualities of ancestors whilst alive, for this determined how they should be approached in prayers.

The Trobriand islanders of New Guinea believe that everybody possesses two spirits. One dissolves soon after death whilst the other, called Balonna, is eternal and exists in another world. Communication is maintained through dreams and trance states. Dreaming of your ancestors is seen by many peoples as a way of preserving contact with the departed. Your dreams provide access to the deeper layers of your being and people today still get helpful information from their ancestors through this means. For example, a woman on one of my courses recounted how her grandmother appeared in a dream and told her to contact a distantly known individual who would have information on a new career opportunity. At the time the person had felt trapped in a very difficult and demanding secretarial job that she desperately wished to leave. Screwing up her courage she called the person and very tentatively explained her situation and the reasons for the call. The individual was just about to advertise a new vacancy in his company, a job that perfectly suited the woman. Needless to say she was successful in her application. It led to promotion and a very rewarding career change.

### Ancestral animal spirits

In some cultures the family ancestors were thought to adopt animal form. The Kwakiutl tribe of the northwest coast of North America believe that killer whales are the spirits of people who have drowned and will protect the tribe. Miwok elder Alice Proutt admonished her grandchildren with the words: *'A bear is just little person. You should not want to eat him, because may be eating your grandfather.'* Similarly, the Zulu peoples of South Africa refrain from killing certain snakes because they think they are the souls of their ancestors.

Uaica, the great magician of the Juruna Indians Brazil, was guided by the jaguar ancestor called Si, who helped him frequently through dreams. This enabled Uaica to perform great magical feats, to carry out all forms of miraculous healing with the touch of his hand and to do much to improve the lot of his people. This lasted until the Juruna persuaded Uaica to marry, one of their maidens, though much against his will. She deceived Uaica by taking a lover who, jealous of Uaica's powers, tried to kill him. Uaica escaped and disappeared forever into a hole in the ground.

Aboriginal myths are interesting in that there is no reference to the ancestors or tribal heroes travelling across the sea to Australia. According to their beliefs they have always lived on their tribal lands, which are especially sacred because of the ancestors. These are perceived as manifesting through different animal species, but most important are the spirits that created the land during Alchera (Dreamtime). It is they who travelled about, shaping the landscape and showing the people how to survive. Their task completed, they subsided back into the earth. Different animals took on the form of tribal ancestral spirits. One of the most popular of these animal ancestors was the lizard, possibly because of its human-like `hand'. Many aboriginal ceremonies are an enactment of the ancestral stories.

# Religious beliefs

### Taoism

In April families celebrate a festival in which they refurbish the tombs of their ancestors. It is a time both to mourn recently lost loved ones and to celebrate family togetherness. Those ancestors who achieved importance during their lives are especially venerated at such times, and their help is sought for the benefit of the family.

Taoist priests also hold special ceremonies to help and appease 'homeless souls', those who have died without being given a proper burial. Around the fifteenth day of August a special ceremony known as the 'Festival of the Floating Water Lamps' is held to help the souls of those who have drowned. One member of the Taoist household carries a lighted candle and places it in a paper lantern or boat, which is then floated downstream as a guide for souls on their upward journey. These ceremonies are especially important for people living near major rivers such as the Yangtze, where thousands of people can drown if a major flood occurs.

The Taoist calendar is divided into three parts, beginning with the Chinese New Year in February. The first six months are called the 'Reign of the Spirits of Heaven'. This period is followed by the 'Reign of the Forgiver of Sins', which lasts three months and begins with the festival of the Floating Water Lamps. The final three months of the year come under the 'Reign of the Water Spirits'. At the end of the 'Reign of the Spirits of Heaven' the gates of hell are believed to open, offering the lost souls of evil and unjust people a second chance for redemption. The living can help these souls by performing special acts of piety or good works, such as giving to the poor. In this way the family can help any deceased relative who had lived a wicked life on earth.

Taoists believe that at death the Shen or spirit remains close to the body until it is buried. The part of the Shen that governs strong passions, such as anger, grief and joy, becomes interred with the body. The immortal part goes on either to a blissful existence or to face punishment from the gods for any misdeeds committed on earth.

## Ancestors and the I Ching

The *I Ching* or 'Oracle of Change' has its origins in the mists of Chinese antiquity. It is not known when the first oracle was cast, but it is thought to date back at least four thousand years. The influence of the *I Ching* on Chinese belief and culture was just as great as the Bible in Judeo-Christian societies, although it expressed very different concepts. It is based on the interweaving of two dynamic forces which were perceived to flow through all aspects of creation. As already stated, these were known as 'yang', which represented an out-flowing masculine force, and 'yin', a feminine, receptive, inflowing energy. These two energies are most famously symbolised by the 'Tao' symbol but they were also expressed through the development stages of the *I Ching*. In this case the 'yang' energy is expressed as a straight line (—) and the 'yin' as a broken line (– –). Within Chinese belief these dynamic forces were seen to combine together to form four more patterns which could be expressed as follows:

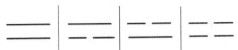

A further stage was developed in which additional 'yin' and 'yang' lines were added to the previous four forming eight possible combinations depicted thus:

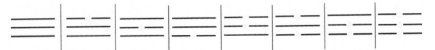

These eight symbols, called trigrams, are perceived to represent eight major archetypal principles.

Symbolically they were considered to depict a family comprising mother and father with six children (eldest son, middle son and youngest son and eldest daughter, middle daughter and youngest daughter) in which the position and type of 'yang' or 'yin' lines is the determining factor. For example the three 'yang' lines is the father, whilst that with three 'yin' lines is the mother. Each family member represents a distinct archetype with its attendant qualities and associations.

Like the original universal classification into either 'yin' or 'yang' energies, the Chinese also categorised all facets of their life under these eight archetypal headings. This is perhaps most widely known today through Feng Shui which involves the placement and orientation of buildings and their contents in accordance with the perceived harmonious relationship of these eight principles. For example the 'Father' archetype called Chien represents the head of all things and finds expression in human activity through rulers, kings, emperors, government buildings, town halls, the chairmen of companies or in the natural world through the tops of mountains, the sun and so on.

These eight trigrams are the basis of the sixty-four hexagrams that form the famous *I Ching* 'oracle'. The hexagrams are formed by the combination of any two trigrams or archetypal principles.

What is so fascinating about this developing pattern is that it mirrors exactly the family tree in its progression backwards through time to the great-grandparents generation. Indeed these yin/yang symbols can be seen as a figurative way of denoting the direct ancestors. For example the father is represented by a single 'yang' line, whilst the mother is a single 'yin' line. Going back one stage to the grandparents generation (two lines), the father's father can be shown as two 'yang' lines, whilst the father's mother can be depicted as a 'yin' line (feminine) over a 'yang' line (father's side of the family tree). On the other side of the tree the mother's mother can be shown as two 'yin' lines. Stepping back a further generation (three lines), your great-grandfather on your father's side can be shown as three 'yang' lines and so on. The chart on page 87 in Chapter 5 shows the position of these symbols in their correct placement within the family tree.

We all have two parents, four grandparents, and eight great-grandparents, making fourteen ancestors back to the third generation. The number fourteen, as will be seen, crops up in other contexts too.

It was the *I Ching* that the earliest emperors consulted when conferring with the ancestral spirits. This oracle and the commentaries upon it by Lao Tzu and King Wen became one of the most important foundation stones of Chinese philosophical thought, and endured for nearly three thousand years. Hexagram 37, The Family, states:

> The correct place of the woman is within; the correct place of the man is without. That man and woman have their proper places is the greatest concept of nature. Among the members of the family there are strict rulers; these are the parents. When the father is in truth the father and the son a son, when the elder brother is an elder brother and the younger brother a younger brother, the husband a husband and the wife a wife, then the house is on the right way. When the house is set in order, the world is established in a firm course.

The idea of the importance of the family to social order was central to Chinese thought. Whilst we might justifiably argue today about the rigidity of the ideas of Hexagram 37, in essence it speaks of the need to find order within in order to establish harmony without.

Another way of looking at this hexagram and its reference to the family would be to see it reflecting the 'family' of the *I Ching* trigrams and their development from the symbolism of yin/yang energies. In this context an integral part of Chinese belief was the recognition of the need to create a harmonious relationship with one's ancestors.

It will be seen later how the *I Ching* can be used to gain access into family patterns. It surely is no coincidence that a culture that placed so much store upon ancestors should have a system like the *I Ching* which mirrors so beautifully the ancestral patterns.

## Shintoism

In Shintoism, one of the main religions of Japan, can be found many similar elements to those of Taoist belief. Shrines are established to ancestors who in life achieved a high degree of spiritual awareness, or displayed great heroism. These places are regularly visited by their descendants who seek help in making their lives happy and prosperous. In times of special need a shaman-priest would contact the ancestor to obtain advice.

The Tamamitsu sect of Shintoism, to which Dr Hiroshi Motoyama belongs (see p.2), believes in ten precepts as expressed in their scripture *Tama no Hikari.*

1. God is the ruler of the myriad spirits.
2. When there is no Self, the voice of the Divine can be heard.
3. Your life and character are the gifts from your noble ancestors.
4. Purify the old transgressions which run through your family.
5. Do not be consumed by sorrow or stricken with worry.
6. In the human world nothing is perfect.
7. When matrimonial harmony is achieved, success in all things follows.
8. Apply yourself to your appointed task without seeking reward.
9. Your position is established by your actions.
10. Idleness summons all manner of demons and evil spirits.

Of these ten precepts, numbers 3, 4 and 7 bear directly upon the importance of the ancestors and the family.

## Celtic belief

Similar ideas to the Chinese Festival of the Floating Water Lamps, which precedes the gates of hell being opened, can be found in Christianity's All Souls' Day. This festival was adapted from the ancient Celtic one of Samhain. The juxtaposition of Christianity and paganism has given rise to Halloween celebrations and belief in the spirits of the dead rising to roam the world on 31 October. In the Celtic festival the ancestors were invoked for their help in providing protection and food for the clan during the year. Since there are few written records about the beliefs of the Celts it is difficult to be sure how much importance they placed upon their ancestors, but in *Celtic Gods and Celtic Goddesses* Bob Stuart writes: 'Underpinning much of Celtic religion is the concept of ancestral descent, or ancestor worship. This should not be regarded as a crude or savage practice, for it conceals a very sophisticated psychology and metaphysics running through all legends and myths, and manifestations of the gods and goddesses, and was interwoven deeply into Celtic society.' The dead found a haven in special locations, such as Glastonbury Tor in Somerset, which then acquired a sacred status. It was at such sites that they could be contacted to bring help to the people and bestow the gift of second sight.

## Christian traditions

As already mentioned, ancestral patterns in Christianity were viewed in the biblical sense of the sins of the fathers. In the Catholic Church and other Christian denominations the souls of the departed are understood to journey to heaven if they have been particularly virtuous, to purgatory if they have led a normal life or to hell if they have been particularly wicked. Only in certain circumstances, where the spirit or soul has died tragically or is greatly disturbed, might it stay around to haunt a place or person. Interestingly, in my work in healing the disturbed energies of places I have from time to time had to release souls who were too terrified to move on — they firmly believed that if they did they would end up in hell.

The Christian dead are firmly ascribed to their allotted station and, although in practice a person might sense or feel the presence of particular ancestors, they are not seen as having any special role in the religious life of the individual unless they had been especially virtuous. However a survey published in the *American Journal of Psychiatry* indicated that 66 per cent of the recently bereaved people interviewed had felt, sensed or had some tangible evidence of their departed relative coming back to comfort them. This is an amazingly high percentage.

## Family history and the Mormons

The Church of Latter Day Saints has an unusual view of the importance of the ancestors and deserves special mention. The Mormons possess the most extensive family history library in the world, which is held on microfilm and is consulted regularly by genealogists studying family history. The family is seen as being both *'eternal and sacred in nature ... Jesus Christ lives and is the Saviour of mankind'*. The ancestors are seen as part of that family patterning and therefore of special importance to the continuity of existence.

In order for the ancestors to obtain eternal life it is necessary for them to be baptized into the Church, which can be done by proxy by the living relatives. Joseph Smith, the founder of the Mormons, stated:

> *'The greatest responsibility of the world that God has laid upon us is to seek after our dead. This doctrine [of salvation of the dead] was the burden of the scriptures. Those Saints who neglect it on behalf of their deceased relatives, do it at the peril of their own salvation.'*

In their booklet entitled *Why Family History?* the Church states,

> *'The sole purpose of this work is to perpetuate family life in all eternity and to gather family members together into the presence of our Heavenly Father, whom we love, honour, and revere.'*

This practice incorporates the belief that the living relatives have the power specifically to help their ancestors.

# Ancestral myths

## Egypt: Isis and Osiris

A myth which appears to give insight into the significance of fourteen main ancestors stems from Ancient Egypt. It is one of the most famous of all Egyptian creation stories and, like the *I Ching,* played an integral part in the belief systems of the Ancient Egyptians. It involves a group of gods and goddesses, the children of the sun god Ra, who came to earth to bring the benefits of civilization, agriculture and craft work to mankind. They were ruled over by Osiris, a wise philosopher king whose consort was called Isis. Having first civilized the Ancient Egyptians, he decided to take his knowledge to the rest of humanity.

Whilst he was away his wicked brother Set plotted to take over Egypt for himself, intending to trick Osiris and kill him on his return. His evil plan began with the making of a sarcophagus that would exactly fit his brother.

When Osiris returned, Set held a magnificent banquet in his honour and then promised to give the sarcophagus to whoever it fitted. Eventually Osiris lay down in the sarcophagus and at that moment Set sealed the lid and threw it into the Nile. He then took over his brother's realm. Isis was distraught and went in search of her husband, finally finding his body. However, before she could bring him back to life Set found the couple and this time cut the body of Osiris into fourteen pieces, which he scattered throughout Egypt.

Once more Isis went in search of her husband and collected up all the parts, except his penis which had been eaten by a Nile crab. She breathed life back into Osiris, but he determined from then on he would rule only from the spiritual realm. It was left to Osiris' son, the falcon-headed god Horus, to fight Set on behalf of his father.

The myth can be interpreted on many levels. It tells of the split between the materialistic side of our nature (Set) and the spiritual part (Osiris). It is Isis (love) that reconnects us to this spiritual aspect within. Yet the number of parts of Osiris when he is cut up (fourteen), and the destruction of his sexual organ, suggest a link with ancestral patterns. Moreover, when Osiris is resurrected it is from the land of the departed that he holds sway; the souls of the dead are brought before him to be judged on the righteousness of their lives in the 'weighing of the heart' ceremony, where the symbolic heart of the deceased is weighed in the scales against the feather of Truth. Those souls that were found to be true of heart were welcomed into the halls of Osiris, the Ancient Egyptian equivalent of heaven, whilst those who failed the test were devoured by the crocodile monster. This belief was a central doctrine in Ancient Egypt, and over time developed into the elaborate mummification rites that tried to ensure the successful outcome for the soul's final journey.

One interpretation of the Osiris myth is that to be whole we must, through love (Isis), reintegrate our fourteen ancestors in a balanced way within our psyche. These patterns, when united and healed, will allow for a new sense of selfhood (Horus) that can draw upon the support of the spiritual realm (Osiris) to help, inspire and guide us.

## The generations of Jesus

The number fourteen crops up on a number of occasions in the Bible, most notably in Matthew 1:17 which reads, in the King James version: 'So all the generations from Abraham to David are fourteen generations, and from David to the carrying away into Babylon are fourteen generations; and from the carrying away into Babylon unto Christ are fourteen generations.' The repetition and emphasis of the number fourteen are interesting. It is known that seven was a sacred number to Judaic peoples, as evidenced by the days of God's creation; but why fourteen? Perhaps it is a coded reference to the three generations of direct ancestors.

## What is the reality of these myths and beliefs?

Myths themselves are naturally open to many layers of interpretation: they speak to us through symbolic language and should not necessarily be taken literally. Whether the Ancient Egyptians believed the Isis/Osiris myth in the same factual way that Christians believe in the resurrection of Christ cannot be determined. What cannot be disputed is that both groups perceived their respective 'sons of God' as powerful forces that could be called upon to aid them in their daily affairs. Invoking the aid of forces beyond the physical world lies at the heart of all religious belief, and in this sense all religions are intrinsically the same. The only difference is the interpretation of who or what is being called upon for help. It would seem possible that our ancestors might have an important part to play in this process.

CHAPTER 3

# *Family Patterns*

Most families have stories of their forebears that get passed down. This is a rich heritage that can shape the beliefs and experiences of developing children and provide a continuity of experience that is embodied within the family structure. This chapter examines the role of family beliefs and traditions in shaping our ancestral patterns.

## Family myths

Many individuals are aware of specific patterns of function, structure or relationship that run through their families. These sometimes become embodied into family myths, and get passed on through stories about previous generations. The way that grandmother tackled a certain situation might be held up as role model for how the family members are expected to act.

Taboos or 'things we don't talk about' create distortions that are easily picked up by young children. Some grow up with an awareness of some dark secret relating to their family. Such issues can often revolve around sex, which until recently was often approached with hypocrisy and double standards. Social attitudes to illegitimacy have inflicted terrible suffering upon some individuals. In Britain in the early twentieth century, for instance, giving birth to a child out of wedlock was regarded as a symptom of mental instability and young unmarried mothers were often incarcerated in mental institutions. Yet in reality most families have had instances of illegitimacy at some stage. Fortunately today such attitudes are rapidly changing, and for more recent generations family stories have probably been superseded by television, which presents more collective human patterns.

## Adoptive families

Patterns of behaviour can be repeated even by adopted children. In her book *Ruth Ellis, My Mother,* Georgie Ellis has indicated some of the parallels between her own life and that of her mother, who had the notoriety of being the last woman to be hanged in Britain for murder when she killed her lover, David Blakely.

Although growing up in an adoptive family where she had all the benefits her mother missed, Georgie displayed many similarities of behaviour. Her adoptive parents wanted her to become a doctor; instead she insisted on a career in modelling, like her mother. She has had three marriages and numerous affairs — one of which could easily have ended the same way that Ruth terminated hers, and was with a man whose initials, coincidentally, were also D.B. However in Georgie's case, despite feeling that if she had a revolver she would have pulled the trigger on her lover, she turned her back on the relationship.

She claims that her book is an attempt to explain her mother's actions. Georgie feels that the spirit of Ruth is still communicating with her, 'from the other side', asking her 'to put the record straight'.

## Unconscious influences

We often play out unresolved ancestral patterns in our lives. The poet, April Ryedale, who had been introduced to the concept of ancestral healing recently wrote:

"I have begun to see how far I have been living my father's life rather than my own in formulating goals and feeling helpless to achieve them. It is only recently that I have attempted to live my own shadow by letting myself into the consuming depression beneath an always bright exterior. I was brought up to understand that the over-protection my siblings and I received as children was due to the terrible accident my father sustained as a four-year-old in 1878 when the family carriage driven by his father overturned, when the horse startled and bolted, throwing out all occupants, killing his mother and leaving him incurably (although at the time invisibly) injured. This in turn prevented him pursuing a military career he had still set his heart on.

Further research revealed that my grandfather himself longed to make the Army his profession, but was indispensable to his father's wool business until he was thirty, and then became a barrister instead. To his self-repressed sternness in not imitating his father's irresponsible philandering (which caused his wife, my great-grandmother, to leave him and emigrate to America) was now added my grandfather's distress at having avoidably caused the family tragedy by driving (against advice) a hunter, not yet properly broken in. I now perceive this as his unconscious metaphor for 'kicking over the traces'. My own father's compulsion both to live responsibly and to live out his grandfather's nature (his father's shadow) led to my brother and me being the bastard children of my father's second serious liaison, when his wife wanted no more children.

My attempts to come to terms, at seventy-two, with living my own life, despite this compulsive and unfinished programme, have been further enlightened recently by reading a letter from my father to Joseph Conrad, whom he knew and admired. In it he asserts his belief that great art arises when it constitutes a vision that the public is just ready to receive. This is exactly my own view as an esoteric poet.

I have in my own self-healing come to see that we cannot (as I have so far sought to do) enshrine a vision of the future if we cut ourselves off from our past roots and cultural inheritance. I thus see my task as seeking to be sufficiently rooted in my acceptance of ancestral connection, yet not so sucked into it that I cannot see and ground the next step ahead, for myself. Creativity is surely a knife-edged business of balancing the old with the new."

## Fears

A fear of specific situations — of water or of catching certain illnesses, for instance — can often be transmitted from generation to generation. One of my clients has a fear of cancer, which sometimes paralyzes her with terror. She is sure that she picked this up from her grandparents, who had frequently expressed their own fears of this disease. Parents' fears are quickly picked up by their children and become incorporated into their own belief structures. Fears surrounding types of physical illness and early death can sometimes be so powerful, and these situations believed to be so inevitable, that occasionally individuals have been known to commit suicide to relieve the pressure of their uncertainty. Whatever the likelihood of some pattern repeating itself within the family, it does not mean that it has to happen: any pattern can be changed if there is sufficient insight and will to do so.

## Changing genetic patterns

In his book *Healing Breakthroughs* Dr Larry Dossey recounts the case of a patient called Max who, in his mid-thirties, suffered a heart attack stemming from a genetic disorder associated with high blood cholesterol levels. Many earlier male members of his family had died at a similar age, so the long-term prognosis did not look good. But Max was a determined individual and his first step was to turn vegetarian and conscientiously to adhere to the different medical regimes for lowering blood cholesterol levels. Unfortunately all this effort resulted in only a small drop in his cholesterol level, and Max felt that he too was fated to die early. But then Dr Dossey prescribed one other method that Max had not yet tried: quiet relaxation techniques. This was meditation at its most basic, simply sitting quietly for twenty minutes twice a day and observing the thoughts entering one's mind and leaving again, without any attachment to them. It worked; ten years on, Max's cholesterol levels have dropped below normal and he holds the longevity record for men in his family. This further suggests the importance of the mind in modifying the patterns that stem from our genome.

One of my students suffers from a genetic defect that causes the ends of the bones to continue growing in a form of tumour. This condition is present in several members of the family on her mother's side. In her particular case it has not been a real problem, since by the time she had reached adulthood the growth had stopped: something within her was able to counteract the defect. Her sister, on the other hand, has not been so fortunate and has had to undergo many operations to remove the tumours. At a superficial level it might seem that one sister was lucky and the other not, yet it could also be that one sister was determined not to let the problem afflict her, whilst the other had a different agenda. Such an affliction has been a means of gaining attention for herself, of helping her feel important in some way.

If this is so, then clearly the genetic defect is not the sole answer to the problem. Something within the mind needs to be healed first. The case of the fishskin boy, described on p.20, shows that is it possible for the mind or consciousness to over-ride genetic patterns. It was perhaps at this level that the monk Rasputin was able to bring some relief to Tsar Nicholas II's son Alexei, who suffered from another genetically transmitted disease, haemophilia.

What these stories demonstrate is that family myths can be changed by simply not allowing oneself to be sucked into believing the inevitability of the pattern. However, some families appear to be particularly fated and have no apparent ability to change the course of the patterns. These families sometimes feel that they have been cursed because of a heinous deed in the past, and such curses have been noted in some of the aristocratic families of Britain.

## Family curses

In his book *Haunted Houses: The Tales of the Supernatural, with some Accounts of Hereditary Curses and Family Legends,* published at the turn of the 19th century, C. G. Harper mentions a number of curses affecting Scottish families. The curse of Moy, the seat of the Mackintosh family, arose when the clan chief murdered the father and lover of a girl from a rival house and forced her to look upon their mutilated bodies. She is supposed to have said: 'Never the son of a chief of Moy might live to protect his father's age. Or close in peace his dying eye, or father his gloomy heritage.' This curse is reputed to have worked until the present head of the Mackintosh clan and his father, who only became chief after the direct line had died out.

The problem with curses is separating prophetic insight from the actual laying of a curse against an individual — something that was quite common in Scotland. One of the most famous of the Scottish prophets was Coinneach Odhar, who lived during the reign of Charles II in the seventeenth century. He is reputed to have accurately predicted the doom of his oppressor's family, the Earls of Seaforth, after the wife of the current Earl had ordered him to be burnt as a witch for divining that her husband was having an affair with a lady in Paris. As he was dragged to the stake he is reputed to have uttered his terrible vision of the future involving the extinction of the Seaforth line. As a sign that his prophecy was being fulfilled he asserted that, of the last four Lairds, one would be buck-toothed, one hare-lipped, one halfwitted and the last would have a stammer. The last remnants of their possessions would be taken over by a white-hooded widow from the east who would kill her sister, and finally the great house of Brahan, the family seat of the Seaforths, would itself be destroyed (Harper, 1899).

Every aspect of this curse came true within 150 years. The daughter of the last male heir, who had returned from India after the death of her husband, had an accident whilst driving a pony and trap that resulted in the death of her sister. The Brahan house was pulled down after World War II.

Another of Coinneach's prophecies ran thus:

*"When Norman, the third Norman, the son of the hard-boned English woman, will perish by an accidental death; when the Maidens [a group of rocks] become the property of the Campbell; when a fox will have young ones in one of*

*the turrets of Dunvegan castle; and particularly when the enchanted fairy flag should be for the last time exhibited; then the glory of the Macleods shall depart; a great part of the estate will be sold to others ..."*

Many years later, beginning in 1799, these prophecies were fulfilled with uncanny accuracy.

Coinneach was certainly an enigmatic character who traditionally gained the power of prophecy at a young age. There are a number of different accounts of how this happened, but in all versions it states that this gift was given to him by the *Sithean,* the ancestral spirits who haunt burial mounds and graves and within whose boundary the gift of 'second sight' lay.

Scotland seems to be particularly rich in these type of stories, possibly because of a strong sense of the supernatural in Scottish tradition, but England also has its share. One of the most destructive curses was laid against the Browne family who, after the dissolution of the monasteries, were granted Battle Abbey in Sussex by Henry VIII. It is said that Sir Anthony Browne gave great offence to the Benedictine monks in ejecting them from the monastery, and the abbot is reputed to have pronounced that they would be cursed *'in sleeping and waking, in eating and in drinking, in all their incomings and outgoings, until fire and water should destroy their house, and should extinguish their family and all their posterity for ever'.* Disaster appeared to stalk the family from that moment, ending in the tragic drowning of the two sons of the last daughter, Mrs Poyntz, in 1815.

The Kennedys in the USA (see p.81) are another family with a reputed curse laid upon them; without doubt they have suffered enormous tragedy, made worse by being in the glare of publicity. There is a legend that the Kennedys had been cursed for some misdeed when their ancestors were living in Ireland. As in Scotland it was just as customary to curse an individual for a misdeed as to bless them for a kindness. However, in the Kennedy family it seems that the most serious disturbances have manifested in the children and grandchildren of

Joseph and Rose Kennedy, the parents of Jack, Robert and Teddy. Another story suggests that Joe Kennedy was cursed, for his anti-British, pro-Nazi propaganda when he was the US Ambassador in Britain from 1937 to 1941. Whether the Kennedys have been actually cursed or whether they are still living out patterns set in motion by Joe and Rose can never be known, yet misfortune still seems to haunt the family.

An article in the *Daily Mail* in the summer of 1996 entitled 'Are the Shand-Kydds cursed?' followed a serious riding accident which broke the neck of William Shand-Kydd. The report highlighted a series of tragedies which have hit the Shand-Kydd family and those associated with them. Such events may have ancestral connections, but we can only be sure when it is possible to establish a clear link in patterning with the lives of other members of the family. Repeating patterns through generations are, almost certainly, of ancestral origin. These can best be tackled through the ancestral healing techniques given in this book.

## Ancestral 'ghosts'

Sometimes deceased ancestors seem to stay in a very tangible way, to look after the family members. A colleague of mine investigating a haunting was aware of the presence of a woman resembling a portrait in the house. This 'ancestor' informed the investigator telepathically that, as long as her portrait was retained, she would protect both the house and the family. When she shared this experience with the family my colleague was informed that there was indeed a legend of this kind associated with this particular portrait. On the one occasion when the family was hard up and had sent the painting to be auctioned, a fire had broken out in the house, as though in warning. Needless to say, the painting was quickly restored to its rightful place; there were no further incidents.

A similar story was told in the *Daily Mail* in Spring 1996. A portrait representing an illegitimate daughter of the Leekes family, called Henrietta Nelson, had been stolen. Always despised because of her origins, Henrietta died in 1815 and was granted her last wish of being buried in the family vault. However, thirty years later her coffin was removed to the local churchyard, after which her ghost is reputed to have first appeared. According to the present owner of the portrait her spirit is now attached to it, and he has warned the thieves that they may have taken more than they bargained for.

## Re-establishing a family connection

Around 1670 the mill on the Dumfriesshire estate of the Jardine family burnt down. Porteous, the miller, was blamed by Sir Alexander Jardine and thrown into a dungeon where he was kept barely alive on very meagre provisions. Sir Alexander left one day for Edinburgh, and inadvertently took the keys of the dungeon with him. On his return he found that Porteous had starved to death, having gnawed his fingers to the knuckle to try to assuage his hunger. From that moment the place seemed to be haunted by his ghost and, despite many attempts at exorcism, the only thing that appeared to keep this restless spirit at bay was the family Bible. The Jardine family fortunes declined and they were eventually forced to leave their home at Spedlins Tower, Lochmaben. Since then the family have moved regularly and many of their business ventures have ended in failure.

The twist to this tale came through the help of the wife of the present Sir Alec Jardine. Mary Jardine is a practising healer and therapist. While giving healing to her husband one day, she suddenly became aware that the ancestral energy from Porteous was sitting across her husband's solar plexus, seemingly still cursing the Jardines. A whole series of psychic impressions followed which strongly intimated that the seventeenth-century Sir Alexander's father, William Jardine, had raped Porteous's mother and that Sir Alexander and Porteous were therefore half-brothers — a fact that was almost certainly known to both of them when Porteous was thrown into prison. Through his neglect Sir Alexander Jardine had been responsible for the agonizing death of his half-brother.

To heal the situation, in 1993 the present Sir Alec consulted a counsellor in Edinburgh who helped him to decide that Porteous and his descendants should be included in the family tree and that in recognition Alec should plant a tree at Spedlins. The agreement of the present owner of the house was given, and in April 1993 the Jardines planted an oak sapling and then read out the first five verses of Psalm 40:

> 'I waited patiently for the Lord; and he inclined unto me, and heard my cry.

> He brought me up also out of an horrible pit, out of the miry clay, and set my feet upon a rock, and established my goings.

> And he hath put a new song in my mouth, even praise unto our God; many shall see it, and fear, and shall trust in the Lord Blessed is that man who maketh the Lord his trust, and respecteth not the proud, nor such as turn aside to lies.

> Many, O Lord, my God, are thy wonderful works which thou hast done, and thy thoughts which are toward us; they cannot be reckoned up in order unto thee. If I would declare and speak of them, they are more than can be numbered.'

Exactly a year later, on Monday, 11 April 1994, Sir Alec became very unwell with a crippling stomach pain; in giving him healing his wife Mary felt there was still a scar left over from Porteous. So they read the Psalm again, and this time felt a complete release for both Porteous and Alec from this mutually destructive influence. Since that time a new optimism has entered the family and a lightening of what was sensed as an unknown heavy burden. The aim has been to free future generations of Jardines from this karmic pattern.

## Family karma and reincarnation

It is an intriguing thought that we may incarnate back into our own families in a subsequent generation. Roger Woolger, author of *Other Lives Other Selves*, who has worked extensively in past-life therapy, is aware that in two of his own lives he was grandfather and grandson in the same family.

Something similar happened to a colleague who had attended one of my ancestral healing courses.

The story started when, during a foot massage, she suddenly shifted consciousness and became aware of a scene in the late nineteenth century. Some young boys dressed in knickerbocker trousers were running in and out of a small corner shop; outside it were some barrels and an old hand-cart. The scene then changed and she saw herself looking over a harbour at a number of three-masted schooners. Then the picture faded.

It meant nothing at the time, so my colleague thought no more about it. Then a few weeks later, when she was meditating, she again shifted consciousness. This time she sensed that she was in a submarine, which she somehow 'knew' was during World War I. Suddenly she became aware of shouting and panic as she 'saw' water rushing into the vessel, at which point she felt that she blacked out. She came out of the meditation feeling much shaken.

A few weeks later something prompted her to ask her father about his childhood. He recounted some details that reminded her of the small boys that she had seen. So she asked whether there was a corner shop near his childhood home. This he affirmed: he and his brother would often go into the shop and, whilst one of the brothers kept the shopkeeper occupied, the other would steal some sweets from the barrel outside. At the time they lived in Bristol and the father confirmed that they often saw three-masted schooners in the docks. She then asked her father about his brother and was surprised to discover that he had died in a submarine during World War I at the age of twenty-five.

Her next experience came from another guided meditation in which she again 'saw' herself in a submarine that was sinking. She had an overwhelming feeling of being trapped in a claustrophobic space and sensed rising panic as the water rushed in. Her first thought was that her soul would be trapped forever in this watery coffin, but then something inside her indicated that she could just fly out. She was suddenly aware that she was looking down upon a scene of wreckage, and noticed four sailors swimming in the sea.

Her father decided to check out the available information on the demise of his brother's submarine, which had been accidentally sunk in the Channel by the British on 15 March 1918. All the reports tallied with what my colleague had 'seen' and experienced in her meditation; the most telling evidence was the four survivors spotted on the surface of the sea.

Clearly what she experienced carried all the hallmarks of someone who had actually gone through these events. It is, of course, possible that she picked up on the memory patterns of her uncle, or that at some level he had conveyed to her what had happened to him. However, the experience was felt exactly as though it was being experienced in the first person, and it would seem more likely that my colleague had lived previously as her father's elder brother.

The final twist to this tale occurred when her father spoke about his brother's wife, who was black and had just given birth to a child when her husband died. Because all the family were against the marriage, she was shunned at the memorial service and afterwards rejected by them. My colleague's father remembered seeing at his mother's funeral a coloured girl of about fourteen, who put some flowers on the grave of what would have been her grandmother. After that all trace was lost of her. However, in the meantime my colleague's daughter had given birth to a mixed race child of part African descent, which she did not feel that she could look after. In the end my colleague adopted that child.

This story would seem to capture a number of important elements within the drama of a family, including the possibility that we might reincarnate into the same family structure. The story also involves a mixed race child as part of the family dynamic, suggesting that patterns keep unconsciously repeating themselves through generations.

In all these accounts and beliefs ancestral influence is strongly acknowledged. Whilst some aspects might seem like superstitious nonsense, the weight of evidence suggests that our ancestors do have an impact upon us, either as souls or as patterns of energy. By what mechanism could our ancestors affect us? Can the dead really exert an influence over the living? To answer this we need to turn to genetics and look at how both orthodox science and some original thinkers are now beginning to view our DNA.

## CHAPTER 4

# Those Elusive Genes

There is no doubt that our genes play an important part in shaping our lives. But to what extent are we the product of that precise chromosome mix that occurred at the moment of conception, and how much is down to other factors? This chapter examines the role of DNA and its recent off-shoot epigenetics, in our lives and its relevance to our ancestors.

From the many studies carried out it is now generally recognized that the heritability of our physical body, such as our height, is between 68 - 84 per cent the result of our genes (Silventoinen et al, 2003), whilst our psychological make-up is only around 35 per cent genetic. For example a Swedish study on depression found a heritability of 42 per cent for women and 29 per cent for men (Kendler, K.S, et al, 2006). This includes traits such as alcoholism, criminality and general emotional responses to situations. Broadly speaking, it can be shown that approximately one-third of our nonphysical patterns come from our genetic inheritance. Within specific individuals this psychological band might vary considerably: some people express many similarities to their parents or grandparents, whilst others display very little. In order to understand the mechanisms through which these inherited non-physical patterns might be affecting us, we need to consider the evolution of genetic studies and what they have to tell us.

## Early work in genetics

The scientific study of inheritance, usually known as genetics, is a fascinating subject that started in the nine-teenth century with the work of the Austrian monk Gregor Mendel. He made a number of meticulous observations on the colour of pea seeds and the height of pea plants.

Sometimes the offspring were quite different from their parents, and these differences could be exploited. The realization that parents contributed to the physical shape of their offspring was known in Ancient Greek times — indeed, at a basic level an understanding of hereditary principles must have been known to early man through the domestication of animals and the development of new strains of crops. But it was not until Mendel's work and that of later geneticists that any understanding of these principles emerged. Early research was based upon repetitive breeding and careful counting for normal and mutant offspring. From these observations the laws of heredity were formulated.

## The DNA molecule

Genetics today is a very different science, based on both chemistry and molecular structures. It began to develop in the 1950s when the DNA molecule was discovered and recognized to be the genetic blueprint found within each living cell. It now involves what is technically called recombinant DNA techniques, but is more generally known as genetic engineering. Individual genes have been isolated, analysed, modified and in some cases 'grafted on to the genes of other organisms. New foods have been developed, DNA fingerprinting is used in both criminal analysis and scientific studies, and possibilities have now arisen for dealing with known genetically transmitted disorders such as haemophilia.

The molecule was first isolated in the early 1950s by Watson and Crick, for which they gained a Nobel prize. DNA is the master molecule of every living cell, conveying information in a precise and well-ordered manner. If it did not fulfil its functions to a very high level, physical life would be impossible. DNA consists of five atoms, oxygen, hydrogen, carbon, nitrogen and phosphorus. These in turn combine to form four separate simple substances called nucleotides known as adenine, thymine, guanine and cytosine (A, T, G and C). The different combinations of these four letters are the codes contained within each DNA chain.

On the surface the DNA appears to have a super-intelligence witnessed most dramatically at the development stage of a foetus. When your parents' sperm and egg cell united at your conception, a process was set in motion that ended up as the amazingly complex being that is you. Consider what happens when this miracle of creation begins. Two separate cells unite, the DNA links up and then the cells start to divide by identically reproducing themselves. But here the miracle really begins, for each cell, although the twin of its brother or sister, 'knows' precisely whether it is to be, for instance, a brain cell, a heart cell or a blood cell, each with its very different functions. Moreover, each cell proceeds to its correct place in this amazingly complex organism.

## The miracle of life

To grasp both the vastness and subtlety of this operation you might imagine a large structure such as the Empire State Building in New York, which stands some 380 metres (1248 feet) high. For simplicity, let us suppose that the entire building is made up of individual segments the size of a house brick. Each segment needs to know whether it is part of the main structure — a floor, a wall or the roof — or part of the fitments such as a light socket, a telephone cable and so forth. Each part needs to fit together in the right way and at the right time for the building to be successfully completed. The finished building must fulfil all its necessary functions and — most importantly — not collapse through structural failure. Science maintains that it is the individual bricks that hold this information, and that the development stages that led to the building were the result of blind chance. However, logic suggests that every building needs an architect or overall plan if it is not to collapse. If this building mirrored the development of a human baby, starting with just two bricks, in the space of about six months a beautiful, unique skyscraper would have been created.

But here is the amazing part. A structure such as the Empire State Building would probably need something in the order of 5 billion individual segments or bricks. The human body is composed of approximately 50 trillion cells, the equivalent of ten thousand Empire State Buildings. This would effectively cover a continuous area of nearly 100 square kilometres or 35 square miles. It is like laying the foundations of all the buildings in central London and finishing them in just over six months. Could the four simple chemical substances of the DNA, the nucleotides, really be the guiding hand behind such a structure? As Dr Deepak Chopra, former chief of staff of New England Memorial Hospital in Massachusetts, states in his book *Quantum Healing:*

> You may find it easy to think of DNA, with its billions of genetic bits, as an intelligent molecule; certainly it must be smarter than a simple molecule like sugar. How smart can sugar be? But DNA is really just strings of sugar, amines and other simple components. If these are not 'smart' to begin with, then DNA couldn't become smart just by putting more of them together. Following this line of reasoning, why isn't the carbon or hydrogen atom in the sugar also smart? ... If intelligence is present in the body, it has to come from somewhere, and that somewhere may be everywhere.

Yet we know from genetic engineering techniques that the genes convey precise information, and are seemingly intelligent. So we are confronted by two problems. First, if the genes are not the source of the intelligence, what is? Second, how do the genes function? Before we attempt to unravel these questions, let's look at how the genes convey information to the body.

## RNA and proteins

To convey its messages to the body DNA replicates itself into another molecule called RNA (ribonucleic acid), which is very similar to DNA but has a few minor changes in its chemical make-up. RNA could be looked upon as the messenger cells of the body, which in turn direct the production of another molecule called a protein. RNA determines the precise nature of the proteins that are produced and could be said to encode the proteins. Not all RNA molecules are involved with the production of proteins, but that is one of their principal functions.

Proteins are the main determinant of an organism's characteristics — whether, for example, it is an ape, mouse or human being. Depending on their function, these substances can be classified into groups, such as structural proteins, regulatory proteins and enzyme proteins. A protein consists of a chain of amino acids, of which there are twenty important biological types. Enzyme proteins speed up chemical reactions in the body by as much as 100 billion times and are highly complex structures that have very specific functions. To turn on a required reaction, such as converting sugar to energy, just one protein, requires a staggering specificity - the equivalent of a key needing a combination of 100 trillion bits to turn a lock. Is it really possible that this level of complexity was the result of blind chance?

Finally, it is known that the genetic information highway travels from DNA to RNA to protein. However, in some cases information can travel from RNA to DNA. DNA is very stable yet under certain circumstances RNA is not, and can be modified by both diet and environmental influences. So the messages relayed from the DNA to the RNA could be changed if the RNA were to vary itself. These messages would alter the way the body would normally respond to certain stimuli. This might be the explanation for the improvements in the boy suffering from `fishskin' disease mentioned on p.20.

To return to the question of understanding the source of our genetic intelligence, we need first to step back in time to understand the origins of current scientific thought on this subject.

## Darwinism

Over the last few hundred years a number of scientists have acquired fame for shaping decades of scientific thought and enquiry. Newton was certainly one, Einstein was another, and in the biological field Darwin must rank alongside them, having given his name to the main theory of evolution. The full title of his most famous work was *The Origin of Species by Means of Natural Selection, or the Preservation of Favoured Races in the Struggle for Life.* This title encapsulates Darwin's idea that evolution is based upon the survival of the fittest. The means were small random mutations of the genes that would on occasion throw up a 'more perfect' model, better suited or better adapted to survival. The process of small, blind, random mutations removed a sense of a guiding consciousness behind evolution. Effectively there was no need to introduce God into the equation and the Christian belief that the world was created by God around 4000 BC, as described in the book of Genesis, could be successfully refuted. The split between science and religion became complete.

This theoretical masterstroke explained all evolutionary developments in simple terms that have proved very enduring. Such was the power of Darwin's observations and logic that subsequent generations of biologists have, with few exceptions, adhered rigidly to these principles. Yet Darwinian theory, despite its many insights, contains some serious flaws which have tended to be ignored.

## Complexity in evolution

The main problem with Darwinism lies in the way that simple systems are considered to evolve to complexity. The simple single-step idea seems attractive until it is tried out against different theoretical models. An example is the notion of how long it would take the random typing of a group of monkeys to produce the complete works of Shakespeare, regarded as being of comparable complexity to the human organism. Mathematically it can be shown that the odds on this happening are so vast as to be virtually impossible.

Another problem that confronts biologists is the production of evidence for the intermediate steps in their evolutionary argument. Clearly changes have occurred within species in response to environmental pressures, yet each of these changes would have to be an improvement in order for the species to survive. If a species did not adapt it faced extinction, which has happened to many creatures and plants throughout the planet's history. But little evidence has been produced for small, single-step mutations; all the data points to much greater evolutionary jumps.

## The eye in evolution

An example of this is the eye, which appears in three distinct forms in insects, mammals and a group of creatures that includes the octopus. The eye is so complex that it has been shown to be mathematically unlikely for it to have evolved through small single-step random mutations, given the length of time that creatures have existed upon the earth. As with the monkeys trying to type the works of Shakespeare, it is hard to see how this can be done, without some form of intelligent design.

This becomes more obvious when one takes as an analogy slide projection equipment, which can easily get out of focus. The fuzzy picture on the screen makes no real sense until it is brought back into focus, which is only achieved by taking large steps; small individual movements lead you nowhere. Only by having a sense that focus is valuable can the necessary evolutionary move be taken. Because of these anomalies the most recent scientific research has started to support the idea of 'directed' mutation, in which the organism modifies itself consciously in response to a problem.

## Fruit flies, rats and blue tits

Mae Wan Ho from the Open University carried out some experiments with fruit flies, in which their environment was changed so much that their long-term wellbeing was seriously impaired. Mutations occurred in the offspring to counter the threat, and fairly quickly a new strain of fruit fly emerged that was perfectly suited to its new environmental conditions. When the environment was put back to what it was before, the fruit flies too reverted to their original state. Yet the next time the environment was changed the new strain of fruit fly emerged almost immediately. This apparent ability to pass on information, contrary to Darwinian belief, has also been observed in other experiments. These changes are now recognised as part of epigenetic influence.

Another fruit fly experiment involved changing the DNA to produce blind fruit flies, and sure enough the next generation were sightless. Yet within a very few generations the fruit flies had regained their sight in response to this environmental impediment. Random mutations could not explain the speed of this change of DNA. Some other factor had to be at work.

A more basic experiment carried out by John Cairns and his colleagues at Harvard involved placing bacteria that were incapable of utilizing lactose in a solution in which there were no other available nutrients. The bacteria were faced with a stark choice: mutate successfully or starve. Not only were they able to do this, but they passed on their ability to future generations.

A more rigorous study along the same lines was carried out by Barry Hall from the University of Connecticut. His bacteria had to perform two mutations in order to metabolize the sugar; this they were able to do, again passing on their ability. The odds on them doing this, in a random way, have been calculated as one in a trillion.

In an excellent summary of the 'directed mutation' debate Neville Symonds, Professor Emeritus of Sussex University, has stated that 'some degree of directed mutagenesis [mutation] ... is an inevitable consequence of how cells function.' Science (or at least some scientists) has now accepted that evolution is not quite the lottery that Darwin suggested.

Another of the main planks of Darwinian theory is that learned abilities from one generation cannot be passed on to the offspring of the next. But this too is suspect. In the 1920s some experiments were carried out on rats which were put through a series of learning tests. Succeeding generations of the original test rats were shown to complete the tests more speedily and — more surprisingly — rats in other countries put through similar tests seemed to start where the original group left off.

This ability to convey information across distances was also noted in the incidence of blue tits pecking through the silver foil of milk bottle tops to get at the cream beneath. The speed with which this phenomenon spread through Britain could not be easily explained by mimicry. It would appear that the technique was independently learnt and also occurred in Sweden, Holland and Denmark. The Dutch case is of particular interest because doorstep deliveries died out during the war years, so many generations of tits were denied this dietary supplement. When peace returned along with the daily pinta, so did the foil-pecking blue tits — as though nothing had happened.

## Lamarck's theory

If Darwin was wrong in suggesting that evolution occurred through small single-step random mutations, are there any other theories that explain these phenomena?

In 1809 the French scientist Jean Baptiste Lamarck published his *Philosophie Zoologique,* which propounded four basic ideas:

- that every considerable and sustained change in the conditions of life produces a real change in the needs of the animals involved
- that change of needs involves new habits
- that altered function evokes change of structure
- that gains or losses due to use or disuse are transmitted from parents to offspring

Implied in these statements are the notions that:

- individually acquired characteristics are transmissible from parents to offspring
- 'intelligent' changes occur in response to changes in the environment

Unfortunately, despite French support the vast majority of scientists have sided with Darwin, and it is the latter's theories that still hold dominance, although modern studies into epigenetics are beginning to change this picture. To understand just how much potentially does get passed down to us from our parents we need to look at recent research into identical twins who have been separated at birth.

## Twin studies

Twins have fascinated scientists for a long time. Comparing identical (monozygotic or MZ, meaning from the same fertilized ovum) twins with non-identical (dizygotic or DZ, meaning from two separate fertilized ova) or fraternal twins gives insights into the extent of our genetic inheritance. Although MZ twins have different fingerprint patterns, their DNA mix is identical since they both come from the same fertilized ovum. They are therefore 100 per cent genetic replicas, and any differences between them must be due to other factors. To assess the extent of these differences identical twins have been compared with non-identical twins. For example, the majority of identical twins are of equal height, compared to less than 50 per cent of fraternal twins. This suggests that height is heavily influenced by DNA.

One of the most intriguing of these studies has been carried out by Professor Bouchard from Minneapolis. It started when he came across an extraordinary story of identical twins who had been separated at birth and were adopted into different families. These twins, called Jim Lewis and Jim Springer, met again when they were thirty-nine and discovered a host of similarities in their lives.

Both their first wives were called Linda; they had both divorced and got married again to women named Betty. Their first sons were called respectively James Allan and James Alan, the only difference being the spelling of Allan/Alan; they both used to holiday on the same beach in Florida; they smoked the same brand of cigarettes; and both had been petrol pump attendants and deputy sheriffs. They had also as children both had a dog named *Toy*, and both had built white benches around the trunk of a tree in their garden. And so the list went on. When Professor Bouchard researched this case he attempted to discover other twins with similar experiences. Since then the similarities in separated twins' lives have been shown to contain many remarkable 'coincidences'.

One set of British twins, Terry Connolly and Margaret Richardson, who had also been separated at birth, discovered that they had both married on the same day in 1960 within an hour of each other. Another set of British twins, Dorothy Lowe and Bridget Harrison, had both chosen to write up a diary for just one year of their lives —1962. Not only did they buy the same brand, model and colour of diary, but when they compared the pages identical days had been filled out. With each separate study the similarities have multiplied, suggesting that there is either a far higher level of genetic programming than was ever previously suspected, or that there is perhaps some 'psychic bond' that links the twins together.

In an experiment conducted in 1994 by *The Clothes Show* on BBC television, three sets of identical twins were sent separately on a shopping expedition, strictly segregated from their other twin for the whole day. From a list of ten shops they were told to choose three and then select from them two outfits. One of the sets of twins, Daphne Goodship and Barbara Herbert, had been separated at birth and had grown up in different families, only meeting again in their late thirties. Like the others in the twin studies they had found many similarities in their lives, yet both were still amazed when they chose two almost identical outfits. Another set, Lucy and Joanne Higgs, had both emphasized the unlikelihood of choosing similar garments because of their different tastes. They were stunned when they both selected leather trousers and a leopard skin top for one outfit and a similar jacket and jeans for the other. However the third set of twins, Peter and Lenny Love, chose different outfits, showing that individual preferences can still over-ride whatever is the link that brings out the similarities displayed by other twins.

Twin studies are taking place in many countries, and the present consensus suggests that a number of personality traits have a genetic component. Neurotic behaviour, which includes phobias and anxiety, is calculated to be 30 per cent genetic, whilst general emotional responses could be up to 40 per cent genetic. A study carried out on 14,000 adopted people revealed that those who had at least one biological parent with a conviction for theft were significantly more likely to commit a similar offence. The story of Georgie Ellis (see p.44) is an example of this patterning.

Other studies suggest that identical twins tend to die at the same time; this can be from old age, illness or, most surprisingly, from accidents. Is there some genetic clock ticking away inside us, ready to stop at a predetermined moment? Or is 'psychic linkage' the cause?

Our genes clearly have a part in shaping our patterns of behaviour and perhaps also in acting as triggers to significant events in our lives. It is tempting to see the genetic material as the primary cause, but there is evidence to suggest that the function of the genes may be somewhat different.

## Intelligence behind genes

In his book Quantum Healing Deepak Chopra goes to great lengths to try to explain the fallacy of seeing the genes themselves as the repository of the body's intelligence. This, he postulates, resides in what he calls the quantum mechanical body, and it is this invisible body that is the true broadcaster of information to the genetic code. He states that 'the mind—body connection [is] like a radio broadcast: mind sending our impulses of intelligence, DNA receives them'. The DNA molecule, then, can be viewed as a complex radio receiving station which picks up different signals broadcast from the quantum realm. This gives us an equation which looks like this:

**QUANTUM MIND ⟶ DNA ⟶ RNA ⟶ PROTEIN**

To support his arguments Chopra has drawn upon the blood cell experiments of Dr Benveniste. Human serum, full of white blood cells, was mixed with goat's blood which triggered the release of histamine exactly as it would in a person with a bad allergy. Benveniste then heavily diluted the goat's blood and the same reaction occurred. This process he repeated until there were no molecules of the original substance left — in effect the 'solution' was just distilled water; but the histamine reaction was set off as before. This experiment was duplicated by other research teams in Canada, Israel and Italy, with the same results. They all found that the body's immune system could be triggered by an antibody that is not there. It appeared that the water held the memory pattern of the original substance, and it was this that set off the reaction.

Now this is exactly what happens when homeopathic remedies are produced. Substances are diluted in water until there are no molecules from the original substance in the solution. The resultant 'mixture' is then dissolved into the neutral base which forms the homeopathic pill. In terms of Western science homeopathy is impossible, yet thousands attest to its effectiveness.

## Resonance

In my book *'The Healer Within'* I tried to offer another explanation of the way that information is relayed from the mind to the body. In an article for Leading Edge magazine physicist Fred Alan Wolf stated: 'The fundamental proposition is that everything is vibration, everything is vibrating. If you can vibrate with it, or attune to whatever it is that is vibrating, a resonance is created. Then you have a way of transferring energy back and forth.'

If resonance is the key to energy or transfer of infor-mation, are there any existing models that can explain the mind/body link? Few people have not been moved at some stage in their lives by listening to a piece of music. It may evoke a memory, or contain a particularly moving sequences of notes, that stirs the emotions and imagination. Why do these resonances affect us so greatly?

Music theory tells us that vibrational energy is transferred when two objects such as two tuning forks are pitched at the same frequency. If one fork is sounded in a room and another of the same note is held nearby, the second tuning fork will start to vibrate. But music theory also tells us that energy is transferred across octaves. So if middle 'C' on a piano is played all the other 'C' notes will start to vibrate as the resonant energy is relayed across the octaves. It is tempting to imagine these octaves stretching into infinity, to realms way beyond the physical dimension in which we live.

Let us suppose that our physical body represents the lowest octave of the piano, our emotional body another, our mental body a third and the spiritual dimension a fourth. We might like to include also another octave representing Chopra's quantum body. When any note is sounded, information will immediately be sent across all the octaves. Any thought or feeling will affect the body and, conversely, substances taken into the body such as alcohol will affect our mental and emotional states. Information will be flowing through us all the time. This is perhaps why we feel an emotional response when music is played. Evidence to support this hypothesis can be found in those unfortunate individuals who suffer from multiple personality disorder.

## Multiple personalities

Many multiple personality cases, now known as Dissociative Identity Disorder (DID) have been documented and carefully studied. What often happens is that the disease patterns of one personality change when another personality comes to the fore. In one case a boy named Timmy presented nearly a dozen different personalities, one of which was allergic to orange juice and made him break out into hives. It happened even if this personality took over whilst the juice was being digested: the physical body suddenly broke out in blisters. Yet when the original personality returned the process would immediately reverse itself and the blisters would begin to subside. When a patient's personality shifts, all manner of illnesses, scars and other impediments can appear or disappear.

Applying these examples to the piano analogy, it is as though another personality takes over playing the top octave of the piano and immediately the lower 'octaves', and in particular the body, resonate to a different tune.

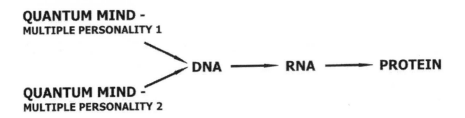

This ability of the mind to impose a physical pattern on the body has also been noted by Dr Ian Stevenson in his detailed researches into past lives mentioned on p.14. In many of these cases where the individual felt that in a previous life he or she had died a violent death, birthmarks on the present body coincided with the former injuries. As with the multiple personalities, it is as though the physical body takes on the resonant patterns from the soul or personality.

## Morphic resonance

Another theory that has gained ground of late has been postulated by Dr Rupert Sheldrake. He suggests that fields exist at a subatomic level which allow resonances to be transferred across space and time. Known as morphic fields, they hold the memories of nature in a similar way that water held memory in the Benveniste studies described on p.66. According to Sheldrake, it is these fields which give shape and meaning to the genetic structure — which propelled the fruit flies into regaining their eyesight after being made blind. Because they hold these resonant patterns, the morphic fields can also transfer information across space so that information learnt in one part of the world is immediately available to species in another. These fields could be seen as a form of non-physical 'super-information highway' holding the memory of everything that has taken place.

This idea has special significance in relation to our ancestors. If, as Sheldrake suggests, these fields hold all memory patterns, then recorded upon them would be the lives of our ancestors. It was stated earlier that, according to scientific theory, energy can only be transferred where there is a resonant connection. There must be global resonant expressions for human beings as well as for trees and other species. Within these fields we will obviously connect most strongly into those resonances that reflect humanity as opposed to those that express 'treeishness' or different animal traits. But at a specific level, because our genetic coding contains our ancestral patterns, these resonances will be the ones that will theoretically and practically have the most profound effects upon us. The formula can then be extended to look like this:

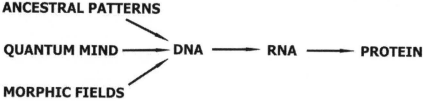

**ANCESTRAL PATTERNS**

**QUANTUM MIND ——► DNA ——► RNA ——► PROTEIN**

**MORPHIC FIELDS**

In this picture you are influenced by three distinct fields from the non-physical level: your ancestors or ancestral fields; your soul or quantum mind; and the primary fields of humanity, which Sheldrake calls the morphic fields.

## Ancestral voices

Have you ever played that game in which two groups of people try to sing different songs, with the idea of getting the opposing team to take up your tune? It requires a great deal of effort and will to focus on the song that you are singing and often just one or two powerful voices can soon pull others into singing their song. I am sure, also, that there have been occasions when, in the company of a strong character, you have felt influenced either beneficially or adversely by their resonant energy. In the same way ancestral information or patterns could be flowing through you; individual ancestors may be singing siren songs that are pulling you into their tune. Something of the memory or habits of your ancestors could well be impacting upon your life.

How you handle this information must inevitably be very individual and will depend on the precise mix of your genetic structure; twin studies (see p.63) show this. The exciting thing is that these memories are not fixed. It is my firm belief that we can go back into this data bank, just as we can access a computer and alter the information lying there. In this way we can heal not only the patterns coming directly to us but also the information for future generations.

In this chapter I have attempted to explain the ways in which ancestral patterns come down to us, and particularly to draw attention to some of the problems of previous gene theory, although modern studies in epigenetics are changing the previous rigid interpretation of the DNA. If we use the radio metaphor there are two potential problem areas. It may be that the radio is itself defective and therefore relaying distorted signals. In this case repairing the radio (repairing or modifying the genes) will bring benefit. Alternatively the programmes coming from the transmitting station may be impaired. In this case, isolating the particular frequency within the radio may be of interest but will not in itself change the seat of the problem. This can only be achieved by dealing with the imbalance at its causal level. Clearly it is possible to change the way that organisms respond by modifying the genetic code, just as we could alter the radio to pick up different frequencies to receive other channels. Medically changing the codes may bring very positive advantages in helping to cure certain genetically based illnesses such as haemophilia. However, as Dr Samuel Hahnemann, the founder of homeopathy, believed, if the cause of a particular imbalance is blocked from its normal expression, the danger arises that it will deepen and come out in a more serious way in a future generation. This is why my preferred approach with the ancestors is to attempt to heal or rebalance the family patterns rather than to try to block ourselves off from them.

For some people this may seem like an enormous or impossible task. Yet in practice it need not be so difficult. There are many ways in which influences can be modified or ameliorated. If this task seems too great, there are also steps that can be taken to de-link from our ancestral patterns — to inhibit the messages coming through to us from this other level. How this can be done will be revealed in Part 2 of this book.

CHAPTER 5

# Setting Up a Family Tree

Before embarking upon healing your ancestral patterns you will need to construct a family chart containing as much information as possible. If you do not have any direct knowledge of your heritage, it is still important to set up a family chart along the lines of the one given on p.75. In one sense it does not matter whether you know anything of the life of a particular grandfather or grandmother, and in any case most people in the West have no more than scanty information about their great-grandparents. It is still very possible to work on balancing the energy patterns that flow down to you from these relatives. Yet gathering information can be fun and often brings powerful insights to the surface. This chapter examines the practical methods that you can use to put the flesh on the bones of your family tree and explains how to gain some initial insights.

## Keeping records

Tracking down family information is fascinating, offering glimpses into the way people acted in the past. Gather as many detailed records as you can, including photographs and any factual information. When working on your family tree from a healing perspective it is a good idea to keep a logbook or diary in which you note down any perceptions that you gain. Into this category also might come any meaningful dreams that you have whilst working on your ancestral patterns. Externalizing information in this way can enable you to see the patterns that are working through you and how shifts are manifesting. Your outer world is a reflection of the inner one. When you change your inner dynamics, your outer world will change too, and noting down any significant events will give you insight into what is happening in your relationship with your ancestors.

Remember that you do not have to have complete records, or indeed any at all, to work on your family patterns. Moreover, healing your family tree can run at the same time as research into your family history.

## Family history

The most important source of information on your family is other members, sometimes distant cousins. Researching family history has become an increasingly popular pastime, and I have been very gratified to discover that some of my own previously unknown relatives have been quietly carrying out their own researches. Try to gather as much information as you can, particularly photographs and old letters that convey a feeling of the life of your ancestors.

Family history is a little different from genealogy or the study of pedigrees, which is more concerned with establishing family relationships and descent. To begin with, you will not need to go back further than your great-grandparents' generation. This includes your father and mother, four grandparents and eight great grandparents, making fourteen primary forebears. To this list could also be added any cousins, uncles or aunts, which help to give a more rounded view of the family patterns, and also any children.

If you are lucky, you may find that another member has already carried out some research. A large number of family histories have been written up over the years, and it is possible that a few enquiries may reveal a lot of information. Families who have emigrated to other countries often have a strong desire to track down their ancestors, and it is possible that segments of your family tree have already been researched. In my own case, a composite family history was completed by some relatives in Australia who traced their descent back to a common ancestor from Britain who lived in the mid-nineteenth century; on the other side of my tree a book has come to light containing a family history from Germany.

You will often need to contact other members of your family, whether known or unknown, to gather as much information as you can. Some people are very good at holding on to old documents and photographs, which can be a valuable source of insight and information. Aged relatives become a rich source of knowledge; even if some of what they say is inaccurate, their perceptions can be very revealing.

Once you have exhausted all the personal avenues for obtaining information you must make a few important decisions. You could accept what you have so far discovered even though there may be gaps. Alternatively you could embark on researching into official records. When I first wrote this book online research was unknown. Since that time websites, such as Ancestry.com or Genes Reunited have sprung up offering detailed information that was not previously easily accessible. This should be your first port of call even if you only sign up for a short period of time you could save yourself hours of research work. You might choose to contact a professional genealogist who will carry out archive research on your behalf; this costs money but can provide a lot more information. Or you could carry out your own investigations, which, if you have the inclination, can be fun. Accessing records offices takes time and patience, and the first step might be to join a local genealogical society.

It is also important to remember that new information can come to light in the most unexpected ways, making the whole process like a detective story that never finishes. On a number of occasions after carrying out some healing work on their family tree individuals have reported being contacted by some relative with whom they had not been in touch for a long time. In one case, on the day she was doing some ancestral healing work a person was contacted by an aunt who she never knew existed. It transpired that they both had an interest in the plays of Shakespeare and Elizabethan England. In another case, just two days after attending one of my courses, an

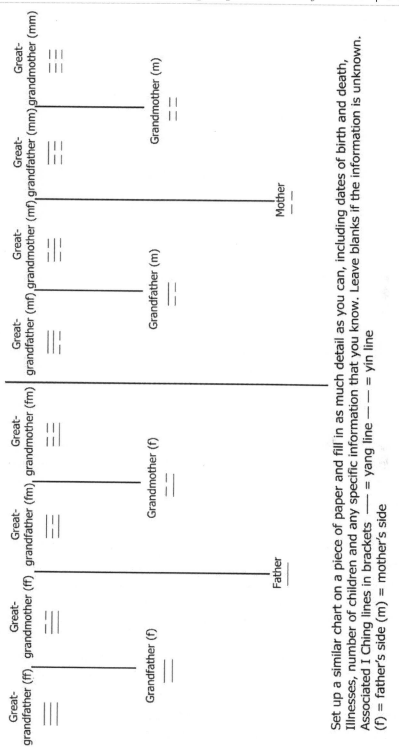

Primary Ancestor Chart

Set up a similar chart on a piece of paper and fill in as much detail as you can, including dates of birth and death, Illnesses, number of children and any specific information that you know. Leave blanks if the information is unknown. Associated I Ching lines in brackets ⸺ = yang line ⸺ ⸺ = yin line

(f) = father's side (m) = mother's side

individual was contacted by a cousin whom she had not seen for twenty-five years. These examples tend to reinforce the notion of a psychic web or energy field that links family members together at a non-physical level.

## Official archives

The next source of information will generally be official records such as birth, death and marriage certificates, census returns, wills and so on. Each country has its own system, but wartime losses mean that the records in some countries are almost non-existent. In the UK National Archives with records of birth, death and marriage are held at Kew, Richmond, Surrey, TW9 4DU. Copies of certificates can be obtained for a small fee.

Another main source of information is the International Genealogical Index (IGI) compiled by the Mormon Church of Latter Day Saints, mentioned earlier. Because of their religious beliefs (see p.39), the Mormons have extensively copied on to microfilm and computer the parish registers from Britain and their equivalent in other countries and these records are held in their central library in Salt Lake City. Copies are held in the local libraries (see list of useful addresses on p.214) of individual countries, and can provide a good starting point for identifying specific parish records. However they exist for births only, rarely mention marriages and never deaths. Most of this information is now available online. Their website is https://familysearch.org/.

## Genograms and family therapy

Once you have drawn up your family tree chart and inserted as much factual information as you can, it is helpful to incorporate some of the underlying family patterns and emotional relationships. The normal way to do this is through a genogram, an idea developed in the late 1970s from a need by family therapists to record family patterns. In their book Genograms in Family Assessment, Monica McGoldrick and Randy Gerson state:

The concept of 'system' is used to refer to a group of people who interact as a functional whole. Neither people nor their problems exist in a vacuum. Both are inextricably interwoven with broader interactional systems, the most fundamental of which is the family. The family is the primary and, except in rare instances, the most powerful system to which a person belongs. In this framework, 'family' consists of the entire kinship network of at least three generations, both as it currently exists and as it has evolved through time. The physical, social and emotional functioning of family members is profoundly interdependent, with changes in one part of the system reverberating in other parts of the system. In addition, family interactions and relationships tend to be highly reciprocal, patterned and repetitive.

The diagram on p.82 shows the genogram for the Kennedy family. On it you will see a number of special symbols that indicate relationships, the sex of different family members, birth and death dates and so on. A full list of these symbols is given on page 78.

Setting up a family tree in this way helps give initial focus to your work. As you proceed with working on healing any patterns, these too can be noted on your chart to provide a reference for the future. I have known cases where people have intuitively felt some aspect of a relationship, perhaps antagonism between two individuals, only to have this confirmed at a later date by another family member.

## Analysis of example chart

If you are suffering a particular problem and you know of at least two other family members with a similar condition, then the origins almost certainly lie within the family tree.

The chart on p.79 gives an example of a genogram back to the great-grandparents' generation. Certain patterns stand out immediately, and those which relate directly to the subject (shown as ME/Millicent Emily) can be listed as follows.

1. Depression: This is the main psychological problem of the client which has its origin in the mother's side, involving

## Genogram Codes

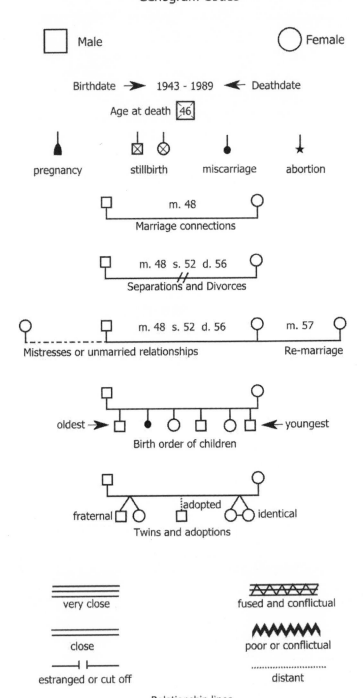

Example Chart

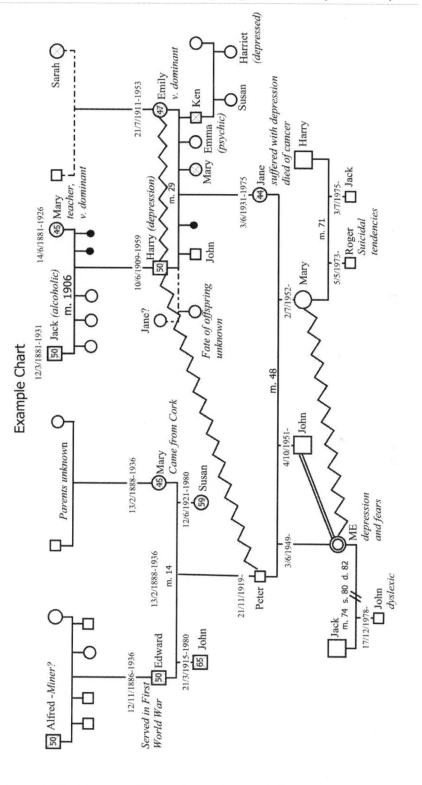

directly the mother, the mother's father (grandfather Harry) and the mother's paternal grandfather (great-grandfather Jack). It has also manifested in a cousin (Harriet) and a nephew (Roger) who has suicidal tendencies. The original problem would appear to stem from the great-grandfather Jack who suffered as an alcoholic. Information on the great-grandmother Mary suggested that she had an overly dominant personality, which may have contributed to her husband's drinking.

The grandfather Harry also married a dominant woman, which led to an affair and an unknown child. There would undoubtedly be feelings of guilt and anger in his relationship with his wife Emily. Whilst Harry was not the eldest child in his family, the client's mother Jane was Harry's eldest child. Eldest children can often carry a great sense of responsibility for the family. The mother Jane was very attached to her father, despite his resentment and conflicts with her husband Peter. No outward conflicts were known around the relationship between the mother Jane and the grandmother Emily although these were suspected.

2. *Names:* A number of repetitions of names appear. The subject married and divorced a man who carried the same name (Jack) as her great-grandfather. Her sister Mary, with whom she was often in conflict, married a man who carried the same name as the father (Harry) whilst her second name was taken from her maternal grandmother.

Repetition of names is a common theme in tracing ancestral patterns, even when family members are unaware of their siblings or ancestors. In the recent case of the writer Lord (Jeffrey) Archer discovering that he had a brother, it transpired that he too was called Jeffrey and had named his eldest son Geoffrey. His unknown half-sister Wendy named her son Jeffrey, though she was unaware of the existence of her two half-brothers. She even used the same unusual spelling.

Patterns such as these indicate the initial areas that should be worked upon. However, it has also been my experience that sometimes other relatives not obviously highlighted come to the fore when intuitively accessing the family tree through the methods given in this book.

## The Kennedy family

The genogram of the American Kennedy family (see p.82) shows many traumatic patterns, with an extraordinary number of premature deaths or tragedies. Four of Joseph and Rose's nine children, as well as the spouse and fiancé of one of them, died before middle age. Rosemary, mentally retarded, had a lobotomy in her twenties; Kathleen and her fiancé were killed in a plane crash just after being cut off by their mother. Ted too was involved in a plane crash, which broke his back within seven months of Jack's assassination; and the Chappaquidick incident, in which Ted was involved in the death by drowning of a young researcher, happened within twelve months of Robert's assassination. Of the twenty-nine grandchildren, one has died of an overdose of drugs, one has lost a leg through cancer, and at least four have been arrested on drugs charges and/or been in hospital with drugs-related problems. There is also a high degree of sexual activity, with many mistresses being openly flouted in full view of other members of the family. Both Joseph's and Jack's affairs were common knowledge, and in recent years another of the Kennedy grandchildren was involved in a rape case.

## The Jung family

Many different types of patterning such as professional activities and careers can run through a family tree. The Jung family genogram (see p.83) shows a link with both the Church and the medical profession. The famous psychiatrist's father, two paternal uncles, all six maternal uncles, his maternal grandfather and two maternal great-uncles were ministers, while both his paternal grandfather, after whom he was named, and his paternal great-grandfather were physicians. In addition, several members of the family believed in the supernatural: his mother, maternal grandfather and maternal cousins Emily and Helena Preiswerk, who claimed to be a medium. Jung attended her séances in his youth.

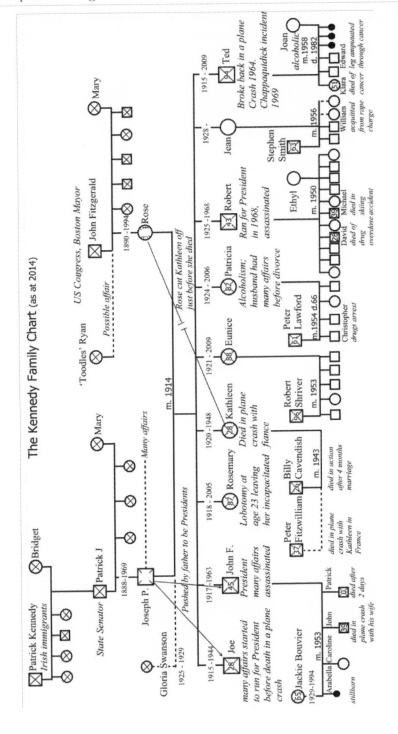

The Kennedy Family Chart (as at 2014)

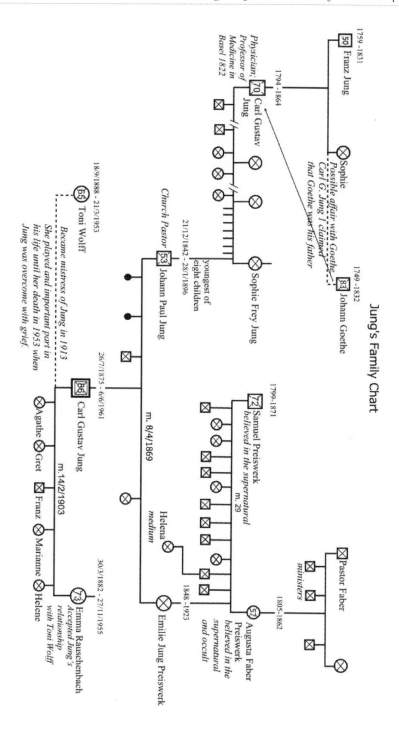

Jung's Family Chart

# Things to watch out for

### Vertical and horizontal patterns

The daughter who has a conflicting relationship with her mother could well find that, if she has a daughter herself, a similar difficulty emerges. If she examined her family tree she might well find that her own mother had the same problem, and so on. Dysfunctionality travels down through families until an individual tries to change the pattern. But family patterns travel horizontally as well as vertically: in other words, they can be found between parents, siblings and cousins of the same generation as well as repeating themselves in successive generations.

### Family position and gender

Families as a whole also carry generalized patterns of function. What this means is that where you fit in a family, your sex, sibling number (first, second, third child and so on) and brothers or sisters all play their part.

First-born children often carry a special feeling of responsibility and over-conscientiousness that can sometimes seem parental. They might indeed have had to take on a minor parental role whilst still a child if they were asked to look after a younger brother or sister. They could also feel that they are responsible for carrying on the family traditions or maintaining family welfare. Youngest children, the 'babies' of the family, can afford to be more spontaneous and care-free. They might well have less respect for tradition and authority. Gender is important too; boys are sometimes (some would say often) given greater attention or seen as more important than girls. A single child will sometimes have been over-protected, or smothered in a way that creates inner tensions. Such children might find it hard to 'leave home' and, even if married, always lean heavily on their mother or father for support or advice.

### Family triangles

The initial relationship pattern of a family will be two-person, the mother and father. But all the research shows that such paired or dyadic relationships by themselves are inherently unstable. A third partner to the relationship will be sought, and this is generally a child. Indeed, within any family relationship a number of triangles can be created, between parents, children and grandparents. Sometimes an outside person, a lover or close platonic friend, will provide that bond. Triangles have a stability about them even if some aspect is in conflict, whilst pair bondings are in themselves much less stable.

### Opposites

'*Without contraries is no progression,*' said the poet, artist and visionary William Blake. Another pattern that is likely to be observed in any family tree involves opposites. It is a fundamental life principle that any extreme of behaviour in one individual is compensated for by its reverse in another. As Jung pointed out, the cosmos seeks wholeness, which means balancing the opposites within any system. For example, one family member may be an inveterate gambler, whilst another will be very prudent or even a miser. Alcoholism and teetotalism are another such duality. The black sheep of a family may be carrying the family's roguishness, which other members cannot own within themselves. If extreme behaviour is manifested by any one family member, always look for the person carrying the opposite; the family saint and the family sinner are but two sides of the same coin. This is why family therapy endeavours to work on the family as a whole rather than as a series of individuals.

Another aspect of opposites involves looking at those areas which are heavily emphasized or held as taboos. The parent who denounces homosexuality may only be hiding his or her own homosexual tendencies. If they cannot own these qualities within themselves, another member of the family, a child perhaps, will end up expressing them.

## The family chart

Your family chart should contain as much information as you can obtain. It can be helpful to classify your findings under the following six headings:[1]

- family structure
- life cycle fits
- pattern repetition across generations
- life events and family functioning
- relational patterns and triangles
- family balance and imbalance

### Family structure

This includes family members, acknowledged relationships, births, deaths, marriages, divorces, separations, remarriages, single-parent households, numbers of children, occupations, siblings with birth order and known illnesses and so on.

### Life cycle fits

This includes the ages when individuals left home, then age when they married, the age when their first children were born, childhood illnesses, early deaths and so on. Anything that seems out of the ordinary should be noted.

### Pattern repetition across generations

This includes scanning the chart for any repeating patterns across the generations in terms of careers, relationships, family structures (illnesses, alcoholism), coincidences of life events such as birth dates and astrological patterns, life transitions, traumas and so on. Jung's family, where there is a high incidence of Church ministers, is an example.

### Life events and family functioning

This includes events happening at similar times within the family: for example the death of a child in one branch coinciding with a marriage break-up in another. In the Kennedy family, Pat separated from her husband on the day of Jack's assassination.

It is worth identifying any particular rhythms on a seasonal basis within your own life, and then checking these back against anniversary dates within your family tree. For example, one client found that she became very depressed during February; later she discovered that it coincided with the death of her grandfather, on whom she had doted, when she was five. Some aspect of her grieving had not been completed and emerged again, as depression, on a seasonal basis.

## Relational patterns and triangles

These can sometimes be difficult to ascertain, but at the simplest level could be described as either:

- easy, close and harmonizing

or

- difficult, distant and disharmonious

The most obvious triangular relationship is between parents and a child, but it can involve other family members, sexual liaisons or platonic relationships. I know of two families where a third, non-related adult lives within the family group. In distorted forms this can lead to sexual abuse between a father and daughter or to over-dominance by the mother of the son.

It is helpful to note where you perceive the triangles within the family group, even if they are not obvious. It should not be forgotten that the ideal triangular relationship of parents and offspring provides, when working well, the most powerful and stable basis for bringing up a child.

## Family balance and imbalance

In the last category the family is viewed as a whole to see where the primary imbalances and balances occur. It requires a feeling for the various patterns that have emerged within your chart. One way to do this is by making a list of the inherent strengths and weaknesses that you perceive in your known family members. These could be categorized under the following headings:

- career
- possessions and money
- love and family relationships
- character strengths and weaknesses
- lucky or unlucky life events
- accidents and illnesses

- secrets and fears

Look for similarities and also for incidents that represent opposites. For example, there might be a pattern of alcoholism in one generation followed by teetotalism in the next, only to be followed by alcoholism again in the third.

## Becoming aware of patterns

One of the most important conclusions reached by family therapists is that simply being aware of the patterns that flow down through your family tree is the first step to changing them. It is as though the very act of becoming aware helps to free locked-up energy.

The concept that being conscious of something immediately changes its dynamic is now an accepted part of quantum physics. It is known, for example, that light can be understood as either a particle or a wave, each displaying very different modes of behaviour depending upon which way it is viewed. The dramatic fall in deaths from TB in the last hundred years has been attributed in part to an understanding of the true cause of the illness. Instead of being a mysterious force that struck down certain individuals, it began to be understood in medical terms and therefore ceased to be so frightening.

Seeing your own patterns will help you focus on those areas of your family tree that need most attention, and can help you reduce the intensity of the energy coming from them. Therefore both the factual research work and the inner intuitive connections play an important part in reframing your ancestral patterns.

## Changing patterns

Recognizing that it is possible to change the patterns that come down through the family tree is a fairly new concept. Only in the last twenty years has it been known that certain types of behaviour could be inherited from previous generations. Studies on criminality, for example, show that this tendency has a genetic basis. In 1995 an important case was brought before the Appeal Court of Atlanta, Georgia: a condemned murderer claimed mitigating circumstances because he was descended from four generations of very violent individuals. It would seem that he was disadvantaged genetically as well as environmentally in his upbringing. If this appeal is upheld it opens the door for many individuals claiming they were only acting out of their genetic disposition and therefore could not be totally responsible for their actions. It is an idea that seriously challenges the basis of the present criminal justice system. Clearly your upbringing is not the whole answer to the pattern of your life; your inheritance too is playing an important part.

Recognizing these transmitted patterns, family therapists have suggested that unconscious behaviour within the immediate family relationships is the primary way in which they are passed on. It is believed, for example, that the dysfunctional parent will unconsciously influence their offspring through hidden messages. Yet twin studies (see p.63) show that, even if twins are separated, incredible interconnections occur. There would appear to be only two ways in which this can be explained. Either there is a powerful psychic/telepathic link that operates at an unconscious level (many of the separated twins did not know that they were a twin), or the coding within DNA is of a far higher order than previously suspected: an order of exactitude, for example, that determines what day you will have an accident or get married. This is a rather startling thought. I suspect that most people would feel more comfortable with the former idea than the latter. And even if the latter case is true it does not work all the time, as the twin studies have shown.

If we view our genetic make-up as a receiving station, picking up signals from some other level outside ourselves and then re-broadcasting its information to the body, we have a way of solving this mystery. This concept allows an element of free will to enter the picture by determining the way that we receive these broadcasts. We do not have to be swayed by the subtle influences from our ancestors, or from the tapes of our childhood experiences. Our consciousness can over-ride these patterns if we so choose. Here lies the possibility of miracle cures, the spontaneous remission of diseases such as cancer that can and do occur in anomalous ways. Nevertheless it is also foolhardy to ignore any discordant patterns that are influencing us.

**Note:** See page 215 for information on downloading a blank ancestor chart.

# Part 2

# *Healing Your Family Tree*

## CHAPTER 6

# Facing the Past

There are a number of different methods that can be used to clear the conflictual patterns, within your own family tree. These will be explored within this section of the book. Before starting it is worth remembering that regardless of when these patterns were laid down in your ancestry they are still potentially active within your psyche. It does not matter that an event happened a hundred years ago — the dynamics of its pattern can still be with you today. The good news is that your subconscious, or rather your 'higher-conscious' mind, is fully aware of the ancestral patterns that are directly affecting you and that this resource be accessed in order to discover and change them.

To make this process more real it is often helpful, whenever you are working on your ancestral family, to try to have a sense of them all being present with you in the here and now. Imagine for a moment that you are sitting together in a room and are able to converse, and share your experiences. For some this may be a disturbing thought, whilst others might welcome the opportunity to chat with their grandmother or great-grandparents. No matter how difficult your family dynamics have been, you should not fear the process of working to clear these patterns. You have the power within you to change what is causing any inner disturbance. Moreover, any deep work can always be carried out with the assistance of a trained therapist if you so desire.

## Methods of healing

Four principal systems are involved, which can be classified as:

- recognizing and acknowledging your ancestral patterns
- inner dialogue communication
- rituals
- energetic healing

Methods of using rituals and energetic healing will be covered in Chapter 8. This chapter will focus on the additional ways of perceiving the patterns that are part of your family tree, and use of the inner dialogues in this process.

## Exploring hidden patterns

Discovering the webs of energy that flow through your life is an important part of any inner journey of self-discovery and healing. As already mentioned, just perceiving a pattern will often free up some of its blockages. It is also important to remember that you cannot change what you are not aware of consciously, so establishing a sense of the primary patterns within your family tree is an essential first step. It may also be that you recognize a pattern within yourself that you suspect has its origins in your family tree, but do not know where to look. This will be covered fully in Chapter 7. Researching your family history through known family members has already been discussed. However, it is also likely that there will be gaps within your family tree relatives of whom you know nothing or from when you can extract little information. There are two main ways to get over this problem.

- external symbolic communication
- inner intuitional communication

## External symbolic communication

This form of communication works through the use of an external symbol or pattern that you observe or create, and which then requires additional intuitive interpretation to obtain its full meaning. Tarot cards are an example: a number of cards could be selected or a reading carried out for each of your ancestors. Divinatory systems such as the *I Ching,* runes, numerology, dowsing (use of pendulum) and the many different card systems can be adopted as part of this approach. This method can best be understood in terms of what Carl Jung called 'meaningful coincidence'.

## Medicine cards

As an example, one of my students, a film director, used Native American medicine cards as a key to understanding the role of her ancestors, the majority of whom she knew nothing about (see http://www.medicinecards.com/). These cards have animal symbols, such as a bear, buffalo and so on, each of which carries a specific meaning. She selected seven cards at random for each of her fourteen ancestors and then looked at their messages in relation to herself. This she did over a fourteen-day period, selecting one ancestor per day during her morning meditation. By reflecting on the cards and trying to sense the dynamic energy that the ancestor represented within her, she obtained a real sense of connecting back into her family roots. Some of these cards indicated harmonious relationships, others highlighted conflicting patterns. When the latter appeared she would consciously try to balance these energies within herself. She also reported that events during her day often mirrored and emphasized the pattern that she had been working on. She found the whole experience enormously enriching and insightful.

On completing the connection with her fourteen ancestors one thing that struck her forcibly, when she looked back at the cards she had selected each day, was the repetition and grouping of specific cards. They seemed to portray patterns that had been handed down through the generations, which often drew attention to her own strengths and weaknesses. Since carrying out this work she has sensed a real shift within her inner and outer world. Some patterns have lifted completely and the dynamic of others changed. Perhaps most significantly, she now feels much more relaxed and able to cope with her very demanding professional work.

### Other methods

To develop the use of symbolic communication you will need to use one of the traditional systems of divination. There are many to choose from as indicated in the lists given previously. It is important that you feel comfortable with the system chosen, so you should spend some time getting familiar with its potential benefits. Another example, drawn from my own family tree work using a number of different divinatory systems, is given in Chapter 9. Further information on this subject can be obtained from my book *Develop Your Intuition and Psychic Powers.*

## Inner intuitional communication

This form of communication works through your subconscious mind to assess the different dynamics or qualities of energy that come down through your family tree. The word 'communication' is used here in its broadest sense, meaning information exchange, and is not just related to dialogue. There are four levels: *kinesthetic, feeling, auditory* and *visual*. These are accessed through simple relaxation techniques coupled with an inner awareness which is somewhat akin to meditation.

To appreciate how this form of information exchange can be used it is first necessary to comprehend the ways that we experience these ancestral energies within our psyches. Energy is transferred when two aspects are in resonant connection. This is a universal principle and applies to all things. The twin poles of your being are your physical body at one end of the spectrum and your spiritual or inner self at the other. The energy within you flows continuously between these two polarities. When you make contact with another person, those parts of yourself that are reflected in that person will open a gateway, which allows energy to be transferred between you. The same thing happens when we connect with our ancestors. Those aspects of the ancestors that are reflected in you, or are relevant to you, will be highlighted when you link to your ancestors.

Now let us look at the four distinct aspects mentioned above. You will find that some come more easily, or give a better response, than others. This is why all four are important, for if one method does not readily work there is always another to fall back upon. Intuitive people will generally find this system easy, whilst others may find it difficult. If you fall into the latter category, try to persist, for the eventual rewards will be beneficial.

### Kinesthetic

This aspect produces physical sensations of heat, cold, tingling and so on, located in different parts of the body. For example, one client used to get a burning sensation in the back of her neck whenever she thought of one side of her family tree.

### Feeling

This aspect produces emotions such as anger or sadness when a connection is made. One client, when linking with an Irish ancestor who lived in the nineteenth century, was aware of an incredible feeling of loss that this ancestor had experienced when her children had to leave home to find work abroad.

### Auditory

This aspect works through inner dialogues. It is as though the ancestor is passing on specific verbal information. An alternative version of this aspect is spontaneous or automatic writing. Both these methods will be explained more fully later in this chapter.

### Visual

This aspect communicates information through visual imagery. Dreams are a form of this kind of communication, but any symbolic inner picture can have a meaning.

Using the above systems of information, you can build up an inner awareness of the way in which you are experiencing the energy from different ancestors. This can be demonstrated through the following exercise. Select one of your fourteen ancestors: my suggestion would be one of your great-grandparents, particularly one whom you do not know anything about. This will mean that your rational mind cannot easily interfere with what you are picking up.

All these exercises are very powerful. I would not recommend you to tackle more than one per day. In my own case I carried them out over several months.

## The Higher-Self

Before starting the exercise I would first like to mention a very important part of the process, which for simplicity I will call accessing the 'Higher-Self' (H-S). Different names have been given to this part of the psyche, such as the 'inner-self helper' but in essence it is an aspect of our being, that has access to the spiritual dimension and also a complete awareness of the patterns of energy that move through us. It is able to access and bring to your attention those elements within you that are influenced or affected by your genetic inheritance and thereby to direct you in the methods that can be used to clear and release any discordant patterning. The challenge from our perspective is the methods we might use to gain a clear communication with this wonderful part of our being. One element that needs to be stressed is that this part will never interfere with your free-will or the free-will of any sub-personality part of yourself. This is why it will not come to our support unless we directly request its help.

The simplest way to view your "Higher-Self" (H-S) is to perceive this as a very wise being that symbolically exists above you in the spirit realm. Normally in yogic tradition it is through the crown of our head or the Sahasrara Chakra that we communicate with the Divine. In a similar way you can imagine this aspect of yourself existing in the spiritual plane and that you are drawing its vibrational energy down into yourself through your crown chakra. I sometimes get my clients or students to imagine the 'H-S' is like the sun shining in the sky and thence to bring a beam of beautiful sunlight down through the top of the head and anchoring it to the light (Soul essence) within you. This latter part should be anchored somewhere close to your heart. Before any inner work a connection should be made to the 'H-S', with a request that links can then be made to any other guides and helpers that might wish to assist you.

## Inner Exercises

The inner exercises suggested within this book are intended to help you access within to gain insight into what needs to be done to heal and balance some of the energies coming down to you from your ancestors. It might be helpful for you to pre-record the information such as is given below and then to play this back to yourself whilst in a meditative state. In this way you can set the pace on what feels most comfortable.

### INNER INTUITIONAL COMMUNICATION EXERCISE

### *Approximately 15 minutes*

**Aim:** *to access the dynamics of one of your ancestors*

- Sit in a comfortable position, preferably with your back straight. Close your eyes and for a few moments consciously relax your physical body, particularly your shoulders. Next focus on your breathing, feeling it becoming both gentle and rhythmical.

- Direct you attention to your toes and feet. Become aware of them and then relax them. Now think of your legs.. slightly tense the muscles and then relax them... think of your back and spine...feel this is also relaxed... become aware of your fingers and hands... relax them... then... think of your arms and shoulders and relax them consciously... think of your neck and jaw and face and sense they are all relaxed and in balance... then bring your attention to rest at the point between and slightly above your eyes... imagine that you are looking inward at that point and then from there to send a thought of peace and balance to the whole of your physical body...

- Imagine or sense that somewhere within you is a tiny flame that represents your inner soul self or spiritual self. It is perhaps best to locate this in your heart area. When you have located it, feel yourself connecting to it. This will ensure that you are linking all aspects of your psyche.

- Next feel a connection to your H-S as suggested above sensing its energy linking through to your inner soul essence and to your conscious mind.

- Think of the specific ancestor to whom you wish to connect. Where does he or she fit into your family chart?

- Become aware of what your physical body is experiencing whilst linking to this ancestor. Does it feel comfortable or uncomfortable? Are you aware of any specific sensations — tingling, heat or cold — in your body? Do you feel any pain or discomfort in any part of your body? If so, does this correspond with any illness that you are experiencing or have experienced yourself?

- Become aware of your feelings. What emotions do you experience when you think of this ancestor? Try to be aware of at least three distinct emotions.

- Imagine that this ancestor is sitting next to you. On which side do they sit? Then ask them inwardly to tell you three things about themselves that are relevant to you. You will either hear inwardly, or you can just imagine what they might be saying.

- Try to visualize or imagine how they might be dressed as they are sitting next to you. What sort of person are they? Now allow yourself to imagine that your relative is an animal (mammal, bird, sea creature or insect). Take the first image that comes to your mind, even if it makes you feel uncomfortable. For example, if the first image or thought is a snake, which frightens you, try nevertheless to stay with that image rather than changing it. Now visualize this animal in an imagined scene. What is it doing? Does it seem contented or agitated? How is it relating to you?

- Next thank the ancestor who is sitting next to you and see them leaving you. Then slowly bring yourself back to full waking consciousness and open your eyes.

- On a piece of paper, write down and draw all that you have experienced when connecting to this ancestor. Think about the symbolism of the animal. What does this animal mean to you? Do you like or loathe it? Or are you indifferent to it? What additional insight does this symbolism bring?

- You may find that you prefer to tackle this exercise in stages, linking first to what you experience kinesthetically, then bringing yourself back to full waking consciousness and noting down what you have picked up before progressing to the next part. If you adopt this approach, make sure you reconnect to your inner light and H-S before moving on.

- When you have completed this exercise, sit and reflect on what you have experienced and understood from this ancestor.

### Inner dialogues

This is an expansion of the auditory level experienced in the inner communication exercise. It can be approached through entering into direct dialogue with an ancestor, or by using spontaneous or automatic writing.

Verbal communication is a very important aspect of human social connection — it is how we pass on primary ideas. But surprising as it may seem, non-verbal communication, through gesture and so on, is also very important. Nevertheless you can gain many useful insights if you can learn to dialogue inwardly with your ancestors. You can enter into direct conversation with your ancestors to appreciate the different facets of the way their life might affect you. They can tell you why they did certain things that might have caused problems both to themselves and to others. For example, in one such inner conversation my grandfather admitted that he had married my grandmother because he thought that she would bring a level of respectability and stability into his life, rather than because he really loved her. This marriage proved very difficult for both of them.

To carry out your inner dialogues, use the method given in the Inner Intuitional Communication Exercise on p.98.

## Automatic or spontaneous writing

Automatic writing is an extension of inner dialogues, except that you write down your questions on a sheet of paper using a pen or pencil and then through your imagination write a reply. For example, if you posed the question by writing it down, *'What was the quality of the relationship between my maternal grandparents?',* then allow your pen or pencil to write a reply, imagining that this was being dictated either by the ancestor or from someone who knew their situation intimately. The sort of reply you might get could be: *'They were a very loving couple but found communication of their feelings very difficult.'* With such a broad question, there is endless scope for variation. The trick is not to let your conscious mind interfere by thinking about your answer but to write down whatever comes into your head no matter how bizarre it seems.

This may seem a little strange at first, but it is a method of by-passing the conscious mind to access directly into the subconscious, which holds the answers. With practice you will find that the writing will take on a life of its own, hence the term automatic, for you will be expressing the perceptions of your subconscious. Before doing any spontaneous or automatic writing you should carry out the preliminary exercise of relaxing and connecting to your inner light and H-S before you begin. Once started you might find a surprising response to some of the questions that you pose.

There is one note of caution that should be heeded using this method. As a system it works exceedingly well when addressed to questions not directly related to yourself, for in these cases the ego is not involved. However in personal questions, to do with your emotional relationships, the answers can be distorted by your ego wishes. For example a question such as 'Will I get into a relationship with Tom?' will be heavily influenced by what you want to happen and your answers will tend to feed back to you what you want to hear. I have known similar problems emerge when individuals have used this method to assess their 'previous lives'. Always treat with very great suspicion any attachments to well-known historical figures for these are traps of your 'ego'.

The ways around this problem are covered in my book *Develop Your Intuition and Psychic Powers.* In all cases use your rational sense to evaluate the written answers. If the reply does not make sense, think about it further, asking your intuitive mind for greater clarity. However, make sure that any evaluation is done after you have received the full message and not midway through because the answers do not make immediate sense. The responses can sometimes be like a modern art painting requiring time to both evaluate and assess their underlying import.

## Your family's dark secrets

In his excellent book *Family Secrets,* best-selling author John Bradshaw, a major international figure in the self-help and recovery movement, outlines the poisonous effects of dark secrets that are held within our family patterns. The book covers the many ways in which our parents unconsciously project on to us their own unresolved issues. These run across the whole spectrum of human emotion, but generally revolve around such difficult feelings as lust, hate, anger and jealousy. The tendency in much of Western society for many generations has been to repress those sides of the human emotional nature that were not acceptable. That which is suppressed or rejected will inevitably be projected on to others, who will then in part carry it for us. Sooner or later, because of the law of polarity, we will be overwhelmed by the very emotion that we sought to deny.

Individuals within the family will take on and express these unresolved aspects, sometimes becoming the family's black sheep.

To make some sense of what might flow down to us from the family, here are the four categories that John Bradshaw lists as toxic dark secrets. The first degree secrets are the most destructive, but even the fourth degree ones might have an impact.

### First degree - deadly (lethal)

- There is always a victim
- Violates the rights of others to life, liberty, dignity of self and personal property
- Usually against the law

#### *Criminal activity*
Murder
Mutilations/torture
Arson
Terrorism, kidnapping, battering/assault
Mugging
Miinchausen by proxy
Satanic cult practices; racial violence
Gay bashing; drug trafficking
Stalking
Burglary/theft; shoplifting; con games

#### *Sexual crimes*
Rape (including marital and date rape)
Incest/molestation
Sexual torture/sadomasochistic sex; child
prostitution/pornography; sexual abuse

#### *Victimization*
Emotional abuse

Psychological abuse, spiritual abuse
Suicide

## Second degree - dangerous (demoralizing)

- Violates one's sense of personhood
- Has life-damaging consequences for self and others
- Can lead to legal violations

### Substance abuse
Alcoholism; drug abuse

### Eating disorders
Anorexia
Bulimia
Binge eating

### Activity addictions
Sexual promiscuity
Multiple affairs; wife swapping, chronic masturbation with pornography
Voyeurism
Exhibitionism; love addiction; work addiction; gambling addiction

### Birth and identity issues
Adoption
Paternity issues; lost siblings

## Third degree - damaging

- Violates one or more persons' freedom
- Violates boundaries
- Involves conscious or unconscious dishonesty
- Damages good name of others
- Blocks family mutuality
- Creates distrust
- Closes communication

### Family enmeshment
Triangles
Covert family rules
Cross-generational bonding
Compulsion to over protect parents
Rigid family roles
Being scapegoated/labelled the 'problem'

### Marital secrets
Hidden anger and resentment
Sexual infidelity
Married when already pregnant
Unemployment (when hidden from spouse)

### Suffering-related
Emotional illness
Mental illness
Physical disability
Denial of death and sickness; clinical depression

### Intellectual/spiritual
Homophobia
Racial prejudice
Religious intolerance Bigotry

## Fourth degree - distressful

- Damage to self primarily
- Guarding the secret depletes energy and spontaneity

### Toxic shame
Fear
Guilt
Anxiety
Depression

### Contextual/cultural shame
Appearance/body
Socio-economic status; educational level
Social awkwardness

Ethnic shame

Spiritual/religious crisis

These lists are not meant to be exhaustive but are intended to give a sense of the types of problem that can be woven on to family patterns. You might like to check these out against your own family members where these problems are known or suspected, noting which category they fall into.

You will probably find that the majority of the dysfunctions within your ancestral family come into categories three and four. However there is quite likely to be at least one case of illegitimacy (there are two known cases in my family tree) and there may be evidence of some family members expressing aspects of second degree and possibly first degree categories. Having an insight into what could be found will help when assessing your own family dynamics.

Having established the different methods that can be used to access into your own family patterns, and also what to look out for, in Chapter 7 I shall focus on techniques for establishing an order for working on your ancestors.

## CHAPTER 7

# Selecting the Ancestors

Before starting on more direct methods of ancestral healing you will need to establish an order of priority for working on each ancestor in turn. This could be followed in a logical sequence, such as beginning with your parents and working back through the generations. Alternatively you might feel more comfortable working first on those ancestors whom you remember or those of whom you have photographs. However, it has been my experience that the logical sequence rarely comes to the fore if you open up to the higher wisdom that comes through your subconscious mind. In retrospect people are often amazed at how appropriate a particular sequence turns out to be when they have left their intuitive self to determine the order.

There are, then, two basic approaches that you can adopt in all aspects of ancestral healing:

- Factual/logical
- Intuitional

Both have their part to play in ancestral healing. Researching official records or obtaining information through family members comes under the factual heading. Remember that family members' anecdotal stories may not be factually accurate; they do, however, provide insights into family members' perceptions of what took place. When information cannot be obtained by these methods, the intuitional approach is the only option. You could use the intuitive methods first and then check using normal research techniques. A number of my students have had an intuitive insight that is confirmed by subsequent events.

## Known patterns within you

In some circumstances you may know of a particular aspect of your life which seems to have an ancestral origin. This might be a pattern of behaviour or a physical illness that has a genetic element. You will need to track this back within your family to gain a sense of where the problem originated, so that you can heal the situation.

In his book *Healing the Family Tree* Dr Kenneth McAll recounts the case of a woman who came to see him consumed by a desire to gouge out her children's eyes. Nothing within her remembered present life seemed to account for this compulsion, but on looking into her family history it was discovered that one of her ancestors had owned a castle complete with a dungeon and a torture chamber that contained implements for gouging out eyes. Suspecting that this might be the root of the problem, Dr McAll arranged for a Eucharist service of forgiveness to be held with his patient present. Straightaway afterwards the woman's compulsion left her, but something even more remarkable also occurred. The patient had an aunt who was suffering from schizophrenia in a psychiatric hospital. At the time when the healing service was held, her mental problem lifted and she seemed quite cured. This aunt had not been thought about as part of the healing process, yet it seemed likely that healing of the source of the problem, the original ancestor, had relieved a trauma that flowed down into lower branches of the family tree.

This makes one wonder why some members of a family should be so affected and not others. It is tempting to ascribe all such afflictions to personal karma, in the sense that the individual is only paying for misdeeds from some previous life. Whilst preferring the notion of personal karma to the idea that God or fate decrees that individuals need to suffer horrendous experiences, I am not sure that this is the only answer. It may be that some people, at a soul level, choose to take on a difficult life experience because it offers them the chance to explore certain aspects of being in a physical body — perhaps as a way of helping to redeem the collective karma of humanity. If the situation is seen in this light, such people need not carry the heavy feelings of guilt often found in those who feel they are repaying a karmic debt.

Dr McAll's client was able to research her family history to obtain a key that helped clear her obsession. Had this information not been available the only approach would have been through intuitive methods. This chapter explores the various intuitive techniques for selecting ancestors to work on, as well as how you might track back through the family when you know of specific problems within yourself.

## Setting up the chart

The first step in the process is to set up your own sample chart along the lines of the one on p.79, filling in as much detail as you can. Remember that it does not really matter at this stage if there are gaps in your information. The first exercise, which will give you a sense of the different flavours or dynamics of energy from each side of your family tree, is as follows. Initially you will only need to work on your fourteen direct ancestors — that is, your parents, grandparents and great-grandparents. In time you might find the need to give attention also to uncles, aunts, cousins and so on.

### BALANCING AND DIAGNOSING EXERCISE
#### *5 minutes*

> **Aim:** *to determine the balance of energies between the two halves of your family*
>
> - Place your family chart on a table in front of you and sit in a comfortable position with your back straight. Close your eyes and carry out the first two stages of the exercise on p.98, making sure that you carry out the body relaxation exercise, connect to your inner light and then your H-S, before moving on.
> - Next, ask within for your father and mother to come

and sit on either side of you, and imagine them there. Note which side each parent sits. Then assess how you respond to their presence, using the four levels of kinesthetic, feeling, auditory and visual. For example: **Kinesthetic** — what physical sensations do you feel in your body when you connect to your mother? What are the differences when you connect to your father? Sensations of tingling, heat, itching should be noted. **Feeling** — what emotional feelings do you get when you think of each parent? Do you feel anger, joy, peace, resentment and so on? **Auditory** — what do you imagine your parents saying to you? **Visual** — how do they visually appear to you? Do they look young or old; dressed as you would expect them and so on?

- Next think of them connected to their respective parents and grandparents so that you are linked through to all fourteen of your ancestors.

- Once more become aware of the quality of energy that comes down to you from these two sides.

- Now imagine a large pair of scale balances in front of you representing the energy from each side of the family. Visualize what is happening to the scales. You will almost certainly find that they are not evenly balanced and tip to one side or the other. The side to which they tip carries the greatest problems from your family dynamics.

- Ask within yourself for the ancestor that most needs help from this side to make their presence known. Ask them to come to the front and stand before you.

- Try to sense what it is that they are holding and what is needed from you to balance the scales.

- Finally bring yourself back to full waking consciousness and note down what you have experienced.

# Intuitive methods of selection

There are a number of intuitive ways of selecting the particular ancestor who needs attention, as described below.

### Inner light

This is a very simple and effective method if you can allow the intuitive perceptive side of your mind to operate. Place the ancestor chart on a table in front of you, or hold it on your lap. Then close your eyes, attune within and sense the link with your ancestors, asking which one needs to be worked upon. Now visualize a blue, white or golden light shining on to your chart and encircling the ancestor in question. You might see this inwardly or, by opening your eyes, suddenly 'see' this light shining on the relevant ancestor. Many people find this a very effective way of bypassing the intellectual mind and highlighting an ancestor whom they had not originally thought about.

### Coins

This method has been adapted from one of the traditional ways of casting the *I Ching*. You will need two coins and your ancestor chart marked with its yang/yin lines.

Attune within, connect to your inner light and H-S, then shake the two coins together and cast them on any flat surface, noting which side they fall which will indicate the generation:

Two heads      = parents

Head plus tail      = grandparents

Two tails      = great-grandparents

Next you need to determine which ancestor. For this you will need only one coin. Toss the coin once for your parents' line, twice for your grandparents' and three times for your great-grandparents'. Tails represent a yang line (—) and heads a yin line (– –). Check back against your chart (see p. 75) to see which ancestor the coins have selected.

For instance, let us suppose that you initially threw two tails, which relates to your great-grandparents' generation. You will then need to toss the coin three times to select the particular great-grandparent. Let us suppose that the coin fell in the order of heads (yin), tails (yang), tails (yang). The *I Ching* system always starts at the bottom, so reading your pattern would be shown as (☲), which is your great-grandfather on your mother's side. Seen another way, the bottom line (first toss) indicates whether this relates to your father's or mother's side of the family; the middle line (second toss), depending on the parent selected, indicates which of the two grandparents; and the top line (third toss) indicates whether it is your great-grandfather or great-grandmother.

In another example, let us suppose that you initially threw a head and tail, which is your grandparents' generation. Next you threw two tosses, which again produced a head and a tail, (yin, bottom line; yang, top line), which would mean your grandfather on your mother's side.

This is a fairly simple method that reflects the way in which the hexagrams are formed within the *I Ching*. Those who have studied the *I Ching* can adapt this method to suit their particular requirements. For example, having ascertained which ancestor to connect to, you could cast a full hexagram to gain further insight into the underlying dynamics. Alternatively, instead of using one coin to find the ancestor you could follow the traditional *I Ching* method of using three coins to determine each line. This gives what is known as moving lines, which can reverse themselves — yang becomes yin, and so forth. If you use this method you might find that you will be drawn to work on two ancestors at the same time.

## Blank card

In the simplest form of this method you will need to make up fourteen cards; the ones that I have found most useful are those used for small card indexes. Cut them in half for ease of shuffling and then write on one side of the card the names (or relationship to you) of your ancestors and any other information that you might feel is relevant. Shuffle and cut the cards, then turn over the top card which will give you the particular ancestor or ancestors whom you need to work upon.

To give more impact to this method you might like to paint or draw the image of each ancestor on one side of the cards.

## Playing cards

Instead of making up your own cards you can use a set of ordinary playing cards. Pick out the twelve court cards (King, Queen and Jack) of each suit, plus the Ace of Spades to represent your father and the Ace of Hearts to represent your mother. The black cards represent your father's side of the family and the red your mother's, whilst the four suits are related to your four grandparents. Their association would be as follows:

**Spades**    father's side: grandfather plus his parents

**Clubs**    father's side: grandmother plus her parents

**Diamonds**    mother's side: grandfather plus his parents

**Hearts**    mother's side: grandmother plus her parents

The King and Queen represent your great-grandparents, whilst the four Jacks are your grandparents. To select the ancestor, shuffle and cut the fourteen cards and then turn over the top card. If you selected the Queen of Diamonds this would refer to your great-grandmother on your mother's paternal side. The Jack of Clubs would be your father's mother, the Ace of Hearts your mother and so on.

## Tarot cards

These could be used in a similar way to ordinary playing cards, but substituting Pentangles for Spades, Swords for Clubs, Wands for Diamonds and Cups for Hearts. Alternatively you could choose from the Major Arcana the fourteen cards that you feel represent your ancestors.

### Dowsing

Those who know how to use a pendulum can dowse for the ancestor or ancestors to be worked on. This method will allow you to refine your information by indicating those ancestors who are having the greatest impact upon your life. You can then select the order in which you need to tackle them. I suggest that you first ask whether you need to work on your parents, grandparents or great-grandparents. When you have determined the appropriate generation go over each ancestor in turn within that group, in order to select the right one(s). When you have your list you can dowse for the order to put them in.

For example, let us suppose that your pendulum gave a positive reaction to your parents' line and your great-grandparents' line. You might then find that the pendulum indicates that you need to work on your mother and your mother's paternal grandfather, as well as her maternal grandmother. These three ancestors could then be put into an appropriate order through dowsing.

## Tracking specific problems

Any of the above methods can be used for tracking specific health or emotional/psychological problems within your family tree. My own preference is always to check what I have found, using these systems, with the Inner Intuitional Communication Exercise (see p.98), attuning to the ancestor that has been selected. I will always finish these exercises by using the symbol of the scales to see how balanced the energies have become. In some cases they will need to be worked upon over a period of months, so do not necessarily expect them to be cleared quickly.

## The next steps

Once you have ascertained which ancestor needs to be tackled first you can use the methods given above to work through the whole list. It does not matter if you find that you are returning to a particular ancestor more than once. This indicates that further work needs to be done to balance and clear any dysfunctional patterns.

The whole process of connecting to, and balancing, the dynamics of all fourteen ancestors does not have to be done quickly, but could be carried out over a three-to twelve-month period. I would not recommend anyone to tackle more than one ancestor per day, and if you adopt this route you will need to check periodically that the energies are still balanced. In any case you will almost certainly find that you will have to spend more time working on some individual ancestors.

CHAPTER 8

# *Resolving Ancestral Conflicts*

A number of common themes have emerged from people who have spent time working on their ancestral patterns. Obviously those qualities which are beneficial to us need not be of concern. It is those aspects of disharmony or disease that get passed on through the generations that are the problem. Every family contains some imbalances: this would appear to be a normal condition of living in a physical world. None of us is perfect, and we each have aspects of imbalance that need to be addressed from time to time. Generally, as long as these imbalances are not too extreme they can be accommodated within the life pattern. It is when they become excessive or violate normal codes of behaviour that real problems emerge.

## What our ancestors need from us

There would appear from working with many individuals, either therapeutically or within a class structure, that there are three predominant qualities or actions that our ancestors require from us. They are to be:

- acknowledged
- understood
- forgiven

Once this base has been established, all other aspects of healing can flow from it.

## To be acknowledged

Surprising as it may seem, one of the most important facets of healing ancestral patterns that many of my students have sensed from different ancestors is the need for acknowledgement. This might take the form of just being heard, as though frustration has built up through lack of acknowledgement.

This seems to support the idea that one of the tasks of our ancestors after they have 'passed over' is to take care of those members of their family who are still alive. In these cases individuals have been aware of an enormous feeling of relief when the contact is first re-established. It is as though the ancestor has been waiting, sometimes very impatiently, for even the barest of acknowledgements.

Not all your ancestors will respond in this way, however, and there will be great differences in the way you experience their impact upon you. In some cases there may even be surprise that any connection has been made, especially where illegitimate children are concerned. In my own family my maternal grandmother was illegitimate and, although she grew up with her mother, the name of her father was not recorded on her birth certificate. When I meditated upon this ancestor, my great-grandfather, I was aware of a real sense of surprise that I had acknowledged and thanked him for helping to give me life.

Sometimes, also, there is a sense of not having completed a task or of having died too early and not being able to support the family. Contact with the ancestor in question can release this blocked energy. A student of mine felt this to be so with her grandfather, and sensed that this was causing some problems also for her living father. After making the inner connection with her grandfather and talking about it with her father there was a real sense of release over her father's fear of death, and a much greater acceptance of all that he had tried to do in his life. Interestingly, once the idea of letting go and trusting had been established, he cashed in all his savings (it was not a huge sum) and divided the proceeds equally between his two daughters. The cosmos responded by replacing the sum exactly, through an unexpected gift that he received a few weeks later.

## To be understood

Understanding is a very elusive quality which shimmers with a mirage of different meanings. Yet to try to understand the underlying causes that have driven an ancestor to act in a particular way also helps us understand similar impulses within ourselves. There can be many reasons why individuals do things that give rise to feelings of guilt and anger. The social and economic climate of their lives might have impelled some to desperate measures. Others might have been caught up in wars, perhaps as soldiers forced to commit acts of brutality or to witness terrible suffering; or maybe as civilians, trapped between warring factions or ideologies, with their livelihoods, homes and sometimes close members of their families taken from them — experiences that would leave indelible marks on their psyches. Such are the patterns that get woven into us.

Even though some unforgivable acts might appear to have been carried out within the family, by attempting to understand them, by connecting to the ancestor we can acquire some fascinating, valuable and healing insights. In one case a man named Michael, working on a relative who had been at the Battle of the Somme in World War I and had then developed into a wife beater, realized the mutual destructiveness of someone locked into their own suffering. This ancestor felt that nobody would understand the intensity of what he had gone through, and consequently became very withdrawn emotionally. Pent-up feelings eventually broke out in the need to inflict suffering on the person closest to him, which was his wife. At the same time the wife, by not being able to connect to that suffering within her husband, had opened the door for it to be inflicted back upon her.

In connecting to these ancestors, Michael realized that all suffering is relative, and that one cannot say that one person's suffering is greater than another's. The resolution for these two relatives was to try to get them to heal the suffering for each other, for by healing another you are actually healing yourself. Michael then understood that to break out of these karmic loops we need to strive not to inflict on others what has been perpetrated upon us.

## To be forgiven

`To err is human, to forgive, divine,' said the eighteenth-century poet Alexander Pope. Following close to understanding comes forgiveness, in whatever way it can be accepted or given. Forgiveness as defined in dictionaries means to give up resentment against another, or to abandon one's claim against a debtor. It has been shown to have powerful therapeutic effects upon the forgiver as well as the forgiven. Within the family tree there is often a feeling that a relative has carried out some deed that cannot be forgiven because it is too terrible. Connecting to that ancestor and bringing forward the need to let go of these attachments can lead to an enormous release.

Even though the relative has passed over, the pattern of that guilt can flow down through the generations; the living relatives then carry the family karma of that situation. But for forgiveness to work it has to be genuine, and to be really effective it also needs to be two-way. In other words, as you forgive an ancestor for whatever karmic pattern they might have set up within your family tree, you need also to ask for forgiveness from any individual whom either you or your family might have similarly harmed, either deliberately or inadvertently. Finally, of course, you need to try to forgive yourself, which can often be the hardest step to take.

A case from Dr McAll's book concerns a woman in her seventies who suddenly developed a violent temper towards her younger sister, with whom she lived. They had been aware that their mother, who was an eldest daughter, had displayed violent outbursts before she died and it seemed that she might have been the cause of the problem. However, on drawing up the family tree it emerged that the eldest daughter for the past six generations had displayed similar tendencies. The cause seemed to lie in an unsolved murder in the family, committed in 1750. From that date the eldest daughter at the time, Elizabeth, had become an alcoholic, drinking herself to death at the age of forty. The subsequent violent temper tantrums down the generations had also spread to the niece of the two living sisters. After a healing service of forgiveness had been held the situation immediately improved for the whole family, and it was felt that a chain of violent tempers had been successfully broken.

## Recommended healing procedure

The following exercise is a general method for healing ancestral patterns, based upon bringing forward the three qualities of acknowledgement, understanding and forgiveness.

### ANCESTRAL HEALING EXERCISE
*Approximately 10 minutes*

**Aim:** *to bring healing and release to the ancestors*

- Gather together any pieces of information, photographs or whatever you feel is relevant, and lay them out before you. You could if you wished set out flowers, incense or any other object that lends a sense of reverence to the scene.
- Spend some time relaxing, attuning within and connecting with your inner light and H-S.
- Ask for help in this healing process from any higher-level power that you believe in. You might say a prayer either inwardly or out loud.
- Attune to whichever ancestor you have been drawn to connect to. Do this by imagining them sitting in front of you.
- Try to sense what it is that they need (acknowledgement, understanding and/or forgiveness) and then attempt to bring that quality to them.
- Thank them for being your ancestor, and then imagine that you are lifting them into the sunlight.

- Sense that any changes in the patterns are flowing down through to you and other members of your family.
- Finish by again asking for help for your relative and thanking whatever spiritual forces have aided you in this work.
- This procedure can be adapted in whatever way suits your spiritual inclination and helps you to feel comfortable.

## Discovering one's ancestors through symbols

Some people find it difficult to gain any clear impressions from their ancestors, particularly if they know nothing about the particular ancestor or are not used to working on an intuitive receptive level. If so, I recommend using one of the many divinatory/psycho-development systems to build up a more complete picture. The main systems, many of which have already been mentioned in Chapter 7, and are described in the glossary, include the I Ching, runes, tarot cards, medicine cards, Sacred Path cards, Angel cards, Olympus cards and so on.

### Healing my great-grandmother

An example of how this might be applied relates to my own great-grandmother Keturah Stacy — my mother's maternal grandmother. All I know about her is that she spent part of her life in the Union Workhouse in Wincanton, Somerset where she gave birth to my grandmother on 26 January 1882 calling her daughter Sarah Jane Stacy. No recorded details of her birth can be traced so it seems likely that she too was born in the workhouse.

In setting up my own family tree chart I chose to use both Olympus cards and Beasts of Albion cards. These, confirming my own intuitions, suggested that she was someone with an idealized sense of love who was swept along by her emotional drives. One of the Olympus cards at I drew for her was the

Gorgon, which stands for confrontation with one's shadow; another was Prometheus, who stole the gift of fire (creativity) from the gods and gave it to mankind, for which he was sorely punished. Prometheus was also cunning in all his dealings. Of the animal cards, both the spider, symbolizing fate, and the dove, representing love and naivety, had been drawn.

When first sitting down to attune to her and send her healing, I drew the Angel card Creativity. There was an initial sense of suffering, bewilderment and betrayal. I then drew the tarot card Justice and the rune of movement, which was reversed, suggesting a blocked energy. I felt that I needed to incorporate a quality of justice into the healing process and to bring forward a balancing of energies between Keturah and the man to whom she had given herself, my great-grandfather. Having finished my healing attunement I then cast the *I Ching* for my ancestor and drew Hexagram 22 which stands for Grace. This is symbolized by fire (again) at the foot of the mountain.

There are many layers to an interpretation of the *I Ching*, but one or two lines from R.L. Wing's translation seem to be worth quoting here: 'The heights of idealism are developing in your personal relationships ... There is nothing wrong in this. Understand, however, that you are now perceiving the most idealistic aspects of love and this is not the basis for either marriage or divorce.' Two additional comments gained from the Hexagram were revealing. The first states: 'If you pay more attention to the vessel than to what it contains, you will entirely miss the meaning of this moment', and the second: 'Simplicity is the path you must take. In this way you will make no mistakes.' Hexagram 22 developed into Hexagram 11, Prospering, which contains the lines: 'There presently exists ideal conditions for new awakenings, healthy growth and progressive plans. ... It is possible now for good and strong ideas to advance the situation while reforming the degenerating elements of the past.' It would seem at least that the *I Ching* was supportive of what had been done!

This example illustrates the ways in which various divinatory systems can be creatively incorporated into ancestral healing. There is no single correct method. You could if you wished use only one system, say the *I Ching,* and carry out readings at different times depending upon which ancestors you are working upon. All these systems will help build up a picture of your ancestor in so far as he or she is impacting upon your psyche. Remember that there are always two elements in this form of healing: the one which your ancestor gives out, and the way you receive that energy. The same is also true when siblings describe their parents, which can occasionally make you wonder whether you are dealing with two entirely different people.

## Healing physical problems

If you need to heal physical illness that has beset either yourself or a relative, try first to go as far back as you can in search of the origin of the problem. Most cases can be dealt with within the three generations back to your great-grandparents. This is because in earlier generations the genetic element will be so diluted that only serious problems will go back that far. However, if you know that your mother, grandmother and great-grandfather all had the same problem, start with your great-grandparent or the earliest generation of which you know.

You will need to send energetic healing, which will be described fully in Chapter 9, but this time focusing upon the physical conditions as well as the mental and psychological nature. It does not matter if the ancestor is deceased for, as has already been explained, there is a sense in which all time is held in the present. When you have sent healing to the ancestor work on down through the family tree to yourself, feeling that at each stage there is a cleansing and improvement in the energy as it travels down to you. It is most important that you do not omit this stage.

## Non-interactive systems of healing

The previous examples are methods in which you are interacting through your imagination with particular ancestors. There are also a number of healing systems in which energy or resonance is transmitted at a distance. Radionics is perhaps the best-known example of this type of approach. A radionics practitioner will diagnose through their meter the origins of a person's imbalances and then broadcast the correct vibrational energy back to them. If a practitioner felt that one of the causes of an individual's problems stemmed from ancestral patterns they could quite easily broadcast the correcting vibration back to that person. But there is also another way in which they could approach this problem.

If the idea that the energy fields of your ancestors are still connected to you is correct, there is surely no reason why the radionics practitioner should not treat the ancestor also. After all, why deal with the effect when you can treat the cause? This type of thinking may seem bizarre, but in theory it should be no more difficult to treat someone through time as through space. Normally radionics practitioners like a physical 'witness', a blood spot or piece of hair, before carrying out their treatment, but I know of some who treat only through the name.

Again, if you are confident about your dowsing skills I see no reason why you should not dowse a particular homeopathic or Bach remedy for an ancestor and then stand that remedy on a card with the ancestor's name upon it. I know of some healers who use this method as a supplement to sending distant healing. They will sometimes place a crystal on a sheet of paper with a person's name written upon it. If it can work for somebody over a distance, it should also work through time.

If you wished to do something similar yourself you could use either a stone or a crystal. Carry out the various steps for attuning to your ancestor, then, in thinking of the healing going to them, imagine that the energy is going into the stone or crystal. When you have spent a few minutes doing this, place the crystal on a card bearing your ancestor's name.

# Healing Prayer

Find a place where you can be quiet and light a candle. Then spend a few moments meditating on your family and the ancestors that have preceded you. Feel a link to your guides and helpers and above all to your 'Higher-Self' (H-S). You might also like to feel a link to the archangel Raphael as Lord of Healing and Karma. Then say out loud the following words.

> *"Through the Power of my 'H-S'; through the light and love of the Father/Mother God and through the Lords of Karma, I connect to all of my ancestors stretching back for seven generations.*
>
> *I acknowledge the power of your influence as it flows down into me and the family karma to which I am bound. I send back to you all love, light and forgiveness; requesting that you too forgive each other – I forgive you, I forgive you, I forgive you.*
>
> *I call on all of your Higher-Selves and the power of the Father/Mother God vested in me, to release any stuck or 'earthbound' influences or any sub-personality parts that may be trapped at the physical earth plane – I release you, I release, I release you.*
>
> *I also ask your forgiveness for any omission or act that I have carried out that does not honour your legacy – please forgive me, please forgive me, please forgive me.*
>
> *I call down God's blessing on our family and all of the members that are contained therein, sending that same thought of love and balance to all future generations that choose to experience within this family that they may be blessed and lead fruitful lives – so be it, so be it, so be it."*

You might like to record these words into a suitable recording device and then have them played back to you, whilst doing the ancestral release meditation.

This meditation should be repeated three times, but I would suggest that this is not done one day after another but spread out over several months, or perhaps a year, allowing different levels of healing to take place in the meantime.

The following exercise can be linked to the Healing Prayer exercise above. I have called this a Temple/Church meditation as it is likely that your ancestors would have been familiar with such a place. For simplicity this inner meditation exercise is structured for a church; it can, however, be any place that you regard as a sacred space. If so you will need to adapt the process to suit your inner reality.

### INNER HEALING TEMPLE/CHURCH MEDITATION EXERCISE
### *Approximate time 5 – 10 minutes*

**Aim:** *to release ancestral karma and send healing to one's ancestors*

- Close your eyes and carry out the body awareness exercise before linking to your H-S.
- Imagine yourself entering into a church and then proceed to the altar end of the church and face the eastern window in front of the altar.
- Call upon God, the Christ Consciousness energy and also the support of the four archangels, Michael, Gabriel, Uriel and particularly Raphael.
- Then turn around and move to the end of the choir facing the nave of the church.
- Now invite into the nave all of your ancestors with those related to your father on your left and to your mother on your right. Have the sense that you are inviting in seven generations of ancestors.
- At this stage send a thought of love, light and forgiveness to all of them and you could also say (or have playing) the prayer given above.
- Then ask whether there are one or two ancestors (perhaps one for each side of the family) that would like to come forward to assist you in healing your family tree. If someone comes forward try and sense who they might be (e.g. from which side

of the family did they come? Are they linked to your grandparents or great grandparent's generation or further back?)

- Ask this ancestor to help you in all future work in healing the family.
- Together with this ancestor stood beside you send a thought of love, light and healing to the whole family.
- Finally thank all those beings that have assisted you and then in your mind lift the whole church, together with your ancestors up into the sunlight.
- Bring yourself back to full waking consciousness and ground your energies.

## Further steps in the healing process

One further exercise involves cutting disruptive threads that are flowing down to you from your ancestors. In addition to sending healing to the different family members, it can sometimes be helpful to cut any psychic links that tie you into the family patterns. This can principally be done with your father and mother, but could also involve other relatives if you felt the need. In carrying out the exercise with each of your parents, imagine that the energy from each side of your family is flowing down to your respective parent. In effect, in de-linking from your parents you are also de-linking from your whole family patterning. I recommend that you allow at least a week between each parent to allow the energies to be properly integrated and to settle down.

However, this method, whilst benefiting you directly, does not deal with the cause of the problem, which lies with one or other of your ancestors. I would therefore suggest that you first carry out the various healing methods on your ancestors before attempting the de-linking exercise.

## EXERCISE TO DE-LINK EMOTIONAL AND MENTAL BONDS
### FROM YOUR ANCESTORS
### *10 minutes*

**Aim:** *to free up the ties of past patterning*

- Adopt your normal meditation posture, carry out your relaxation exercise and then connect with your inner light and your 'Higher-Self'.
- Next think of the parent with whom you wish to cut the ancestral links and imagine that they are sitting in a chair opposite you.
- Connect to them at their highest level: to do this, you can imagine that there is a light above and between both of you. Visualize a golden thread linking you to this light and down again to your parent. In that way you will still maintain your spiritual link with the ancestral patterns, which will allow a new dynamic to emerge.
- Imagine that there is a cord of energy linking your solar plexus to that of your parent. Some people with whom I have worked have visualized this as a rope, whilst others have 'seen' it as chains, a thick log, an umbilical cord or an iron bar. Your subconscious mind will present the most appropriate symbol for you to work on.
- You will need to cut this image, thereby cutting its energy link. To do so, use whatever symbol is most appropriate in relation to how you imagined this energy to be. For example, if you visualized it as a rope, a sword or sharp knife would do. Keep cutting in your mind for as long as you feel the energy is held. It might take several strokes of the sword or knife before the rope is severed.
- When it is cut, imagine that you are absorbing the loose end back into yourself. Then send a thought of healing to help the other parent absorb their end within themselves in a balanced way.

- Next, imagine that you are within your own sphere of light and they are within theirs — two separate individuals who can now relate to each other in a new way.
- Finally, carry out the forgiveness exercise described on p.120 and thank that individual on behalf of your ancestors for all that they have taught you.

With deep-seated cases you may need to carry out this exercise on a number of occasions before the links are finally severed. It will not mean that you are disconnecting from the ancestors completely — only that you will be changing the pattern of how you relate to them.

## Healing rituals for your ancestors

### The use of ritual

Rituals are a very simple way of setting up inner links to bring about change. The story related in Chapter 3 of Sir Alec Jardine planting a tree for the miller Porteous is a classic example of a simple yet very effective healing ritual. The primary need in carrying out a ritual is to be sincere about what you are doing. As long as the ritual is approached in this way, it will be successful. Rituals have played an important part in religious practice throughout recorded history. They can be performed as a one-off ceremony or, like the Catholic mass, repeated regularly in identical form by people throughout the world. They act as a focus for the mind in invoking spiritual or psychic energy or in sending out energy for a specific project, and repetition can have the effect of building up greater focus of mind-power. Many people find it much easier to meditate within a group than on their own at home. This is because a dynamic of energy is created within the group which helps each individual achieve a greater depth in what they are doing. The repetition of a ritual produces the same result.

This section will look at the different ways in which rituals can be used to help connect to your ancestors and bring about change.

## Daily rituals

In the Far East in particular, many people start off their day by saying prayers to their ancestors and asking them for help and protection. In the West few people begin their day with prayers, although some might spend a little time meditating. If you fall into this latter category or you devote part of your day to some form of inner spiritual work you might like to incorporate a thought for your ancestors. This could be done either individually, selecting a different ancestor each day or collectively by sending a thought to the whole group.

One little ritual that I have adopted, particularly when working on healing different aspects of my ancestral patterns, uses a combination of my set of ancestral cards, a healing stone and an Angel card. At the beginning of my morning meditation I light a candle to my ancestors, then shuffle the fourteen cards with the names of my different ancestors on them. After this I cut the cards and select one which becomes a focus for the day. I then draw an Angel card and place it together with the selected ancestor card and a special stone from the island of Iona. (For example, on one particular day I drew a great-grandfather called Carl Bardili and the Angel card Purification.) I then spend a few moments thinking of that ancestor and the quality expressed by the Angel card before moving on to my normal meditation practice.

When interviewing Drukchen Rinpoche, who is one of the high Lamas of Tibet tracing his descent through the divine being Avolokitsvara, for a magazine article, I asked him how long he recommended us to mediate each day, his reply was *'No more than five minutes.'* He went on to say, *'People are crazy and meditation can make you more crazy.'* The implication is that we do not need to spend long hours each day meditating; far better, he said, to spend five minutes in concentrated thought than fifty minutes in mindless drift. Human beings tend to be creatures of habit, so it is often helpful to set aside a regular time for this type of work each day. These daily rituals therefore need not take up a great deal of time — but always go for what seems comfortable for you rather than feel that you have to stick to a set formula.

So if a daily routine of thinking about your ancestors seems too difficult you can just carry out this ritual when you feel the need. Once you have established the idea of wanting to connect to your ancestors, with the intention of freeing any blocks, you will be naturally drawn to thinking of them at appropriate times. If you feel these promptings it is important to act upon them, for they indicate what needs to be resolved. If, for example, you started to think about a particular relative for no apparent reason, this probably indicates a need to connect to that ancestor. Sitting quietly and thinking of them, or carrying out one of the healing techniques already described, will generally be all that is necessary.

## Annual rituals

In the Catholic and Anglican Church, All Saints Day is celebrated on 1 November which coincides with the Celtic festival of Samhain. The day after is known as All Souls Day. This was first instituted as a festival in the monastery of Cluny in France in 993 AD. The story goes that a pilgrim returning from the Holy Land was driven by storms onto a rocky coast near Sicily. Here he found a hermit who told him that nearby was a cavern that led down into the underworld, from whence emanated the cries and groans of the many tormented souls in purgatory. The hermit also heard the screams of the devils when redeemed souls were taken from them through the pious actions and prayers of holy people. They were especially enraged, he said, against the abbot and monks of Cluny. On his return, the pilgrim related what he had heard to the abbot of Cluny who thereupon appointed the day after All Saints Day to be remembered in his monastery as All Souls Day when special prayers could be offered up to help the dead escape from purgatory into heaven. This practice quickly spread to other monasteries and became an established part of the Christian calendar.

This story illustrates a deeply-held belief within the collective psyche of humanity, that people could intercede for, and help, the souls of the deceased; for as a concept it is found in many widely divergent cultures.

Following this tradition, 2 November would be an appropriate time for honouring your ancestors. In Chinese tradition the death dates of the various ancestors would be honoured or celebrated in some way. Making a list of the anniversary dates of your ancestors, where known, can be a good first step in this process.

### Burial rituals

The graves of the ancestors were always considered to be sacred places in Eastern cultures. The graves of our own deceased forebears can be visited and simple meditations carried out in their honour. In the East it is traditional to clean the graves at least once a year as a mark of respect to the ancestors. The graves of our deceased relatives can sometimes hold a great focus of energy because of the emotions of all the people who gathered there when the burial took place. Laying flowers on the tomb can be a way of bringing peace to the past.

However, with the growing popularity of cremation people are less likely to associate any particular place with their forebears. Nevertheless it is still possible to create an area dedicated to them in your garden or some other suitable place. Doing so also incorporates the idea of connecting to the sacredness of the earth that gives us sustenance. But in dedicating such a place it is important to appreciate that it is only acting as a focal point for your connection to your ancestral energies. Even in real burials the spiritual aspect of the soul is not tied to the body in a literal sense but exists in its own sphere of experience.

This chapter has focused on some of the main ways in which you can begin to heal imbalances within your family tree. Traditional native wisdom suggests that we should seek the help of our ancestors throughout our lives. Once you have sensed that any difficult patterns have been cleared, this other-level family connection can go on feeding positive energy into your own life. There is no set time limit on how long it will take to clear all the dysfunctional dynamics from your family tree. The initial work can certainly be carried out in a relatively short period, although more deep-seated patterns may only change as we ourselves shift and grow. In this sense it can become a lifelong adventure that you share with your ancestors, so that when the time comes to leave this earthly sphere you have many friends waiting to greet you.

## CHAPTER 9

# *Energetic Healing*

Before embarking upon the methods that you can use to send healing to members of your family tree, I want to explain briefly how and why healing works. Healing could be described as a form of energy exchange that helps someone achieve better balance or wholeness. Within conventional medicine this exchange usually involves medication, but in practice any exchange — whether it be through homeopathy, osteopathy, aromatherapy, counselling or spiritual healing — that has the specific intention of helping someone achieve wholeness can be regarded as a healing discipline. According to Einstein's theory of relativity, matter and energy are interchangeable. This chapter focuses specifically on a system that involves non-physical energy exchange. In broad terms this system has been described by a number of different names such as spiritual healing, Reiki healing, psi-healing, Christian Science healing, hand-healing and 'energy' healing. Whilst individual procedures may vary between these methods, in each type the mind is utilized to channel and focus some form of power to help or speed up the healing process of another person.

## Healing principles

### Resonances

Let us first look at how consciousness links into the body. As has been stated, there is a growing body of information, particularly from near death experiences, which supports the notion that some aspect of our being can detach itself from the physical shell. Traditionally this part has been known as the soul, but you could equally call it your higher consciousness, inner essence or whatever term you feel comfortable with. The bottom line is that it survives the death of the physical body and indeed continues to exist in another realm of consciousness. It is this aspect that presents itself as an ancestor and which I believe can continue to exert an influence upon the living relatives.

We could say, then, that there are two polarities to the spectrum of your energies that is you: the physical body at one end and your spiritual self at the other. Every other facet of who and what you are lies between these two poles.

One way we can view this idea is to see it as a stepping down in consciousness from the intelligence of your soul to the intelligence of your physical body. Another way, mentioned earlier, is to liken yourself to a piano, on which the bottom octave relates to the physical body and the top octave to the spiritual self. Every other aspect of who and what you are — your emotions, mind, ego, subconscious and so on — lies somewhere in the keys between. When any note on the piano is played, the resonances set up in the string that is sounded cause every other similar note to vibrate: if you play middle C, for instance, every other C note starts to sound. This is a very useful metaphor: it indicates that if we think a thought, its energy is immediately conveyed to all aspects of the self. Science tells us that when two things are in resonant connection, energy flows from the stronger to the weaker. In other words, if there is an energy within you that is creating disease (dis-ease), you will need to generate a more powerful force to change that pattern. Fortunately for us the body generally has very powerful built-in self-healing mechanisms, and if left to its own devices will usually correct any imbalances.

Just as different resonances vibrate within you, so can they be broadcast to others. Most people know the experience of being in the company of someone else and starting to take on that person's emotional feelings. Some people's moods, their feelings of anger, sadness or happiness, can be very infectious. Similarly you might have been thinking about someone only to bump into them in the street or to have them unexpectedly telephone you or send you a letter.

These are all situations in which resonating information is being exchanged between you and someone else. But such information is very subtle, and your conscious mind will usually block out most of it.

## Healing through space and time

In his book *Clairvoyant Reality,* Dr Lawrence LeShan talks about two levels of reality. One is tied to the known physical world, complete with all its scientific laws and principles — in other words, the world as it appears to our physical senses. The other realm operates on a much subtler level and incorporates very different principles: here time and space, for example, create no barriers. This is something that healers have long maintained, since it is the only possible explanation of the fact that healing energy can be successfully transmitted to someone at great distance with apparent no loss of effect. By simply thinking of someone you connect to them, even though they may be a thousand miles away. There are many cases on record of individuals being powerfully aware, through a feeling or sensation in their body, of an accident that had occurred to a member of their family, even though that person might be on the other side of the world.

Extensive anecdotal evidence and research supports the idea that space is no barrier to these healing energies. But what of time? My own work and that of Dr McAll and others attests to an ability to heal the past in a way which suggests that the past is not fixed either. Perhaps a better way of viewing past events would be to see them as concurrent energy fields that hold the thoughts and actions of those from the past. What has been created by thought can also be changed by thought — in other words we can interact with these energy fields through our consciousness, and in consequence alter the patterns of energy that they contain. If we can heal individuals in the present and across space, there is no reason why we cannot heal the past, and in a curious way perhaps the future also. This is borne out to a degree by theoretical physics, for all the main equations work just as well with time going forward as with time going backward.

In his book The Emperor's New Mind, Roger Penrose, Professor of Mathematics at Oxford University, states: 'All the successful equations of physics are symmetrical in time. They can be used equally well in one direction in time as another. The future and the past seem physically to be on a completely equal footing. Newton's laws, Hamilton's equations, Maxwell's equations, Einstein's general relativity, Dirac's equations, Schrodinger's equation — all remain effectively unaltered if we reverse the direction of time (Penrose, 1989).'

It may seem that you are following a particular path that has inevitable consequences, but if you change the patterning that led to that path you will change your future also. The road that you tread would then be in a process of being continually modified by your thoughts and actions. Following this line of reasoning by healing the patterns that come down to us from our ancestors, we will heal both the present and the future.

Doing so will have the effect of removing those impulses from the past that incline you in a particular direction. Using our musical metaphor again, let us suppose that one of your ancestors records a particular tune from their piano on a continuous-circuit tape that repeatedly replays itself long after they are deceased. Depending on how closely your piano is attuned to theirs, you might well find that their tune starts to impose its sound on you, particularly if it has been played with vehemence. Interacting with your ancestor's recorder will allow you to stop the tape and change the tune to one that suits you better.

The following section has been adapted from my book *The Healer Within,* which describes different healing techniques in detail and is recommended to the reader. However, the information given here is sufficient to start the process of healing your family tree as well as to send healing to your own living family members. Healing can always be given provided that you yourself are in a reasonably healthy state.

## The gift of healing

The power to heal is a natural gift that we all possess to a greater or lesser degree and, like all gifts, can be developed with practice and patience. There are many circumstances, such as accidents or illnesses of friends or members of the family, in which healing energy can speed recovery. It is also very effective in helping to maintain a balance within young children and adolescents. I normally send a thought of balancing healing energy to my children every day, and I feel it makes an enormous and ongoing difference to their development. It need only take a few minutes, and they do not have to be present or even aware of what is being carried out. The positive effects — their alertness, speed of recovery from illnesses and general disposition — are very noticeable in their lives.

There are many professions, such as nursing, counselling, teaching and all kinds of complementary therapies, in which the understanding and use of healing energy can be a powerful adjunct. The most important aspect is a desire to help others; second to that comes a belief that healing energies can flow through you. It used to be known as faith healing, which is perhaps a fair description — except that it is principally the healer who needs to have the faith, not the patient.

## The underlying philosophy

There is no one way to heal — indeed, there could be said to be as many ways as there are healers. It is interesting to experiment to discover the method that suits you best, whether it is holding your hand close to an injured area or just thinking of the healing flowing from you in your thoughts. One of the greatest assets of healing can be a recognition of the important link between the spiritual self and the body, and of what needs to be done to bring these two aspects into balance.

All healing should be an offering to assist another individual find balance within. At no time should you try to impose your will on others. Of all the gifts that we possess, probably the greatest is that of free will. It should be respected at all times.

You should approach your healing from the point of view that you are balancing the whole person — body, emotions, mind and spirit. A useful phrase that many healers use is to affirm within: 'Thy will be done.' This covers both the inner spiritual will of the patient as well as the more orthodox belief in the 'will of God'. The spiritual-self within the ancestor will determine how best to use the quality of energy that you have to offer. If you then sense the need to direct your energies to the specific problem as part of the healing treatment, you can do so in the knowledge that you have set up the right safeguards.

## Localised or general healing?

Repeated studies carried out by the Spindrift organization in Salem, Oregon suggest that healing is much less effective when it is only focused on the manifestation of the illness. In other words, if a person receives healing for, say, a heart condition and the healing is only directed specifically to that organ, it has been shown to be between two and four times less successful than if the healing were sent to the whole person. You need to focus on bringing balance to the totality of the individual, whatever you sense that to be. This is an important point when sending healing to your forebears; it means that you do not have to 'know' what their specific illnesses or ailments might have been.

You also need to learn to trust that the higher aspect of yourself will forward the correct healing energies for the ancestor. In one sense all that is necessary is to open up to the healing power and just let it flow through you, trusting in its efficacy. At a more advanced stage, particularly with those who dedicate themselves to healing as a profession, you might reach a point where you become more consciously aware of the different qualities of healing energy that are flowing through you. You will then know, in a conscious way, why you are drawing upon particular forces and what it is that you are doing. When this occurs it is a very exciting moment.

## Sources of healing energy

Once you have decided that you want to send healing to an ancestor, the next important matter is to understand the origin of your energy. There are two primary sources to draw upon. You can either use your own energies or you can connect into reservoirs of energy outside yourself and thus become a channel for that energy.

When healers first embark upon giving healing they tend to draw upon their own energies. The disadvantage is that you will very quickly deplete your system and feel totally drained. This is an uncomfortable feeling when it happens. The key is to learn to act as a channel for healing energies and not to draw upon your own reserves.

Try to keep it simple. Some powerful sources of energy include the sun, the earth, religious figures such as Christ or the Buddha, trees and crystals. In practice the list is endless. Each source of energy will give a slightly different flavour, so to begin with it is better to use the broadest, most general source that you feel comfortable with, as this will give you the best results. If you are religious you could link with God or Allah, in whatever way you understand that force to be. For those who find difficulty with this concept, I would suggest that you think of the sun. Its energy covers a wide spectrum, and at a basic level is the source of light and life within the solar system. There is no restriction on what can be used: one healer whom I know imagines that she is connecting herself to the electricity circuit for her energy — and it works!

With practice the adventurous healer can learn to channel an ever-wider range of frequencies. Healing energy has distinct 'flavours', and in this sense is very different from electricity. For example, an ancestor who appears very angry and aggressive would need a different quality of energy from one who seems depressed or lethargic. Initially you need not worry too much about these differences, although some ideas on how you can project different qualities of energy, by using colour rays and symbols, is given on pp.145-154

There is no set time limit for giving healing. The general rule seems to be to give the healing for as long as you feel necessary. The fastest healer I ever witnessed was a Russian parapsychologist named Barbara Ivanova, who would direct her healing energies for as little as fifteen to thirty seconds. Barbara worked on the principle that she was putting energy into the body, and experience had taught her that she could focus a large amount of energy very quickly. Too much energy being sent into the body can make a person feel very uncomfortable — hence her restriction to a maximum of thirty seconds. Conversely, I have seen healers giving healing for as long as an hour if it felt comfortable. I normally give healing for as long as I can hold my attention on what I am doing, which might be between five and ten minutes. This is quite adequate when sending healing to your ancestors.

## The application of healing energy

Healing can operate in three different ways, to:

- put energy into the system
- balance what is already there
- remove unwanted energy

Many student healers feel that they are not being successful unless they are pumping a lot of energy into their client, but this may not always be necessary. If we go back to our piano analogy, problems occur when the piano gets out of tune. This causes blockages in the flow of energy and disharmony in the sound of the piano. Some notes may only be slightly off-pitch and can very easily and gently be brought back into harmony by adjusting the tension in the tuning pegs. Alternatively some part of the piano might have become damaged through being mistreated, in which case repairs requiring a lot of energy would need to be carried out. Finally, dirt and grime could have encrusted the strings, causing them to sound off-key. The dirt needs to be removed before the piano gets back in tune. In a similar way you can learn to use the power of your mind to balance the energies of your ancestors, remove energies that should not be there, or put energy into the system to repair damage.

Balancing energies generally requires very little effort. Surrounding a person in a thought of peace or love will have that effect. If unwanted energies become caught up within a person, they will need to be drawn off to bring about the healing. At a physical level, viral or bacteriological infections are a form of inappropriate energy where a type of invasion has taken place. Invasive energies can occur at every level: take, for instance, crowd hysteria, when the power of emotion becomes so strong that individuals can be sucked in, causing behavioural activities at odds with their more rational instincts. Sometimes individuals feel they have picked up some disturbed force within their energy fields. Clearing or cleansing these energies is a very important part of the healing process. Finally there are those situations, when directing positive energy, in which considerable power may be needed to repair damage that has occurred at a physical, emotional, mental or spiritual level. The principal question that all healers should ask themselves is 'How can I help this ancestor or person find balance and harmony within?' Remember that the same principles apply even though your ancestors are no longer present at a physical level.

The very act of giving healing to an ancestor or another person will help balance your own energies. It is always a two-way process. This can sometimes take the form of highlighting the part of yourself that requires attention. It is therefore very important to be open to receiving help yourself, particularly if some part of your life has got out of balance. Never be too proud to ask for assistance.

Physical problems are usually the result of imbalances on a mental, emotional or spiritual level. If you are suffering a genetically based illness, or you know that such illnesses run in your family, try to track these back to their source — the ancestor who set up the pattern in the first place. You will then need to send healing to help correct all the previously mentioned levels within him or her.

## Healing procedure

Attitudes in healing are very important. The healing should be offered with 'love', without any sense of imposing it upon the recipient. In dealing with my own ancestors I have never found any resistance to their receiving help in this way. There will always be a subtle connection between healer and client that is not obvious on the surface. The same applies when sending healing to your ancestors — in fact more so, for you are already energetically connected to them.

The steps suggested here form a general guide which can apply to all forms of healing. It has been specifically adapted with the ancestors in mind.

1. Relax and then attune to your spiritual self (light within) and your 'Higher-Self'.
2. Attune to the ancestor and their inner light.
3. Link to the source of healing energy, e.g. Christ, God, the sun, the cosmos or the earth.
4. Direct your thoughts to balance the whole of the ancestor's energy fields.
5. Send healing to any specific parts, e.g. an arthritic knee.
6. Balance the whole person again.
7. De-link from your source of energy and from the ancestor.
8. Sense yourself balanced within, and close down.

The simplest way to send distant healing to one of your ancestors or to any person is to imagine or sense that they are seated in front of you. You do not have to visualize them in great detail for the healing to be effective: just having the feeling that they are there will be sufficient. You should sense the healing energy flowing through your hands, directing itself to your ancestor. When you have finished, imagine that you are lifting your ancestor up into the sunlight, and send a thought of thanks for the help that you have received.

Here is a simple healing exercise that you can safely use to send balancing thoughts to one of your ancestors. Before starting the healing, rub the palms of your hands vigorously together for a few moments, then hold them a few inches apart and imagine a ball of energy held between the palms. Note down any sensations that you feel. It is quite likely that you will experience similar sensations in your hands whilst sending out healing energy.

### ANCESTOR HEALING EXERCISE

*Approximately 15 minutes*

**Aim:** *to send healing to one of your ancestors*

- Select one of your ancestors. Let us suppose that your grandfather was asthmatic and eventually died of pneumonia; the asthma would most likely also have had a psychological element.
- Sit in a comfortable position, preferably with your back straight. Close your eyes and for a few moments consciously relax your physical body, particularly your shoulders. Next focus on your breathing, feeling it become both gentle and rhythmical; then link to your H-S.
- Imagine or sense that somewhere within you is a tiny flame that represents your inner spiritual self. When you have located it, feel yourself connecting to it. This will ensure that you are linking all aspects of your psyche.
- Imagine or sense that the ancestor to whom you are going to send healing is seated in front of you.
- Sense that you are connecting to their spiritual self. To make this more real you could imagine that you are linking the light within you to the light within them by means of a golden thread. Affirm within the words, 'Thy will be done.'

- Connect to your source of healing energy, for example the sun, and feel its energy flowing down through the top of your head and through your hands to your ancestor.

- Sense or hold the thought in your mind that this energy is balancing their whole being (body, emotions, mind and spirit). To make this more real you could imagine a pair of scales superimposed over them. Hold the thought until you sense the scales are balanced.

- Allow your imagination to prompt you to any other aspect that needs healing in a specific way. (In the sample case you would focus the healing energy to the area of their chest to help the asthmatic condition.)

- Return to sending healing to the whole person, but this time imagine that they are surrounded with a halo of light (blue, white or golden — whichever feels comfortable).

- See, in your mind's eye, your ancestor being healthy and well, and then feel their balanced energy coming down through the generations to yourself.

- Disconnect the golden thread that you have been holding between the two of you, and disconnect also from the source of energy that is flowing through you.

- Sit for a moment, sensing that you are balancing your own energies, before opening your eyes.

- If you wish, you can write down your experiences. Keeping a journal can be a helpful device for monitoring your progress in healing your ancestors. Some healers also like to wash their hands after each case and this too can be a useful discipline, symbolizing the de-linking of the energy.

In principle these methods can also be used to send healing to friends, members of your family, pets, plants and other people. There is no shortage of applications for this energy, and it will deepen your understanding and insight to know that you can make a positive contribution to the wellbeing of others.

Healing the ancestors is a very important part of your process of inner development. I have sent healing on many occasions to ancestors, as I feel that some of them need considerable help. It has been a fascinating experience helping to heal members of my family tree, the majority of whom I never met and some of whom I know nothing about; yet I sense their presences all around me. If you wish to pursue a more active role in healing it is prudent to contact one of the healing organizations whose names and addresses are given on p.214. They all run full training courses in this field.

## Colours in healing

As a powerful adjunct to sending healing to your ancestors, imagine that you are directing colours. Healing energy is not like electricity, with its uniform patterns, but more akin to music with its many flavours and nuances. Some music excites us whilst other melodies calm and soothe us, lifting us to heights of emotional experience that may be hard to re-create in any other way. Healing can act in a very similar fashion. Mentally directing different colours or symbols to someone carries the same kind of quality as hearing different types of music.

When sending a ray of colour to an ancestor you will need to imagine that it is coming from your hands and surrounding them with its light. To do this first think of the colour that you wish to generate. It might be helpful having different coloured papers in front of you and to focus on the selected colour for a few moments. Then close your eyes and carry out all the procedures already given for sending healing but this time imagine that you are generating a coloured ball of energy (depending upon the colour selected) between your hands before sending it to your ancestor. Direct it to the area of imbalance. If you have difficulty visualizing a colour, hold in your mind the thought: 'I am using a white [blue or whatever] ray.' Alternatively imagine the colour over the top of your head and feel that you are drawing the energy through yourself before sending it to your ancestor.

There are four main colour rays that can be useful to your ancestors, depending upon what you are trying to achieve; these are white, blue, pink and gold. For a more complete list, covering all conditions, see *The Healer Within*. With practice you might find other colours emerging. If so, try to assess what particular quality they represent so that you can call upon them again. The colour rays can be used singly or in combination, and in any treatment you may need to work with different colours in turn.

## White ray

Although white contains all the colours of the spectrum, it has a distinctive flavour of its own. It possesses an ability to highlight situations, showing where imbalances lie. If you surround an ancestor in white light and use the symbol of the scales, you can ascertain the cause of any problem. Simply ask in your mind: 'Is the problem on a physical level?' and observe what happens to the scales. Your subconscious mind will access the correct information and feed this back to you through the symbol. If the scales remain balanced, you will know that the cause does not lie at a physical level. You can then ask within: 'Is the problem on an emotional level?' and again observe what happens to the scales. They will tip to one side or the other when you hit a problem area.

The white ray carries a protective strengthening energy and incorporates the emotional quality of joy. It can also be used in those situations where an ancestor has felt battered by disturbed energies around them. Surrounding them in an imaginary white bubble of light will help greatly. We all have an energy field enveloping us which has become known as the aura. This extends out from the physical body and, like the earth's atmosphere, is densest close to the physical and more diffuse the further away that one moves. In practical terms imagining the aura extending up to two feet from your body and then surrounding it with your chosen colour will suffice. Like the earth's atmosphere, if the aura is depleted, then its ability to ward off harmful energies is greatly diminished.

Sometimes, when working on your ancestors, you will process a great deal of information while you are asleep. When this happens, you can wake feeling almost as tired as you did before you went to sleep. If this is your experience, imagine that you are building a bubble of white light over your own solar plexus when you lie down before going to sleep.

## Blue ray

An electric- or sky-blue ray represents harmony, spiritual love and cleansing. It is the ideal colour in all cases where the quality of forgiveness is paramount. Blue can be used where family conflicts have occurred and reconciliation is needed. Its balancing quality will help in all cases of genetically based illness and it can be used for washing through and harmonizing the auric energy fields. It is also the most appropriate colour to surround your ancestor at the end of the healing treatment.

## Coral or pink ray

This is a warming, soothing ray and should be used for the relief of pain and headaches and in the treatment of such complaints as arthritis. It is also an excellent ray to use when you sense that your ancestor is in an agitated emotional or mental state. In these cases the ray should be directed to those areas that reflect the particular condition. With mental agitation this should be to the head, and with the emotions to the region of the heart or solar plexus. It is a ray that reflects the wonderful peace and calm that is seen in statues of the Buddha.

## Gold ray

This is a very powerful ray that reflects the energy of the sun in its positive or yang aspect. Circling all your ancestors in a golden light will help unite and balance their combined energies. It has a very protective quality that is excellent at counteracting negative, chaotic or evil forces. It needs to be used sensitively, as some people can find it overwhelming.

# Symbols in healing

Acting in a very similar way to colours, symbols can be used as a psychological aid to connecting to specific energies. Within the development of the human psyche, symbolic images come closest to the language of the deepest part of the self. This is why dreams are predominantly pictorial rather than linguistic. Symbols can take many forms, as our dream world demonstrates, and they carry both a personal and a collective meaning. In healing they can be used in three ways:

- to act as a focus for healing energy
- to pick up information about specific ancestors
- to gain insights into ancestral problems and situations

Over millennia certain symbols have been used repeatedly as representations of particular qualities of energy and have become embedded into the collective psyche. The following exercise on the quality of love will give you an idea of what is meant by this, before we turn to the significance of the individual symbol.

### HEALING EXERCISE

#### *Approximately 15 minutes*

**Aim:** *to send 'love' to one of your ancestors*

- Sit comfortably in an upright chair, or cross-legged on a cushion if you prefer. Your back should be straight. Close your eyes and for a few moments focus on your breathing. Feel it is gentle and relaxed; then link to your H-S.
- Next think of the quality of 'love'. What does it mean to you? Let your mind visualize the answers to the following questions.
- Which colour do I associate with 'love'?
- Where would I locate this quality within my body?
- What animal do I associate with 'love', and where is that animal in relation to me?

- What flower do I associate with 'love'?
- What item of clothing do I associate with 'love', and what do I feel when I wear this in my imagination?
- Now think of someone dear to you, and project your thought of love towards them.
- Now think of an ancestor who you feel needs the quality of love, and send them a thought of love.
- Finally send yourself a thought of love, thinking particularly of those aspects that you dislike about yourself.
- When you have finished, bring yourself back to waking consciousness and open your eyes.
- You might find it useful to write down what you experienced, how you felt emotionally, and what symbolic images came up.

An important point about symbols is not to reject what comes forward. Beginners will often say, 'I didn't like that animal, so I changed it for another.' The deepest part of your being will communicate important messages through symbols to your conscious mind and so can become an enormously rich source of inner wisdom and knowing. Learn to interpret the symbols, not to reject them.

If you carried out this exercise correctly you would have found a number of different symbols coming to your mind, reflecting the energy of love. What these symbols would have told you is how you relate to that particular quality. To link with this energy in future you could draw upon the same symbols and that flavour of energy would flow through you.

The following are a group of symbols, like the colours described above, that are most relevant for ancestral healing.

### Sun disk

This symbol carries a powerful expansive energy that incorporates all the symbolism associated with the sun. It is invigorating and protective and will help you link with the spiritual side of your nature, dispelling fear and doubt. It is said by some to be the predominant ray that Christ used within his ministry. Its all-encompassing quality makes it a very good energy to call upon when starting to learn healing. Many cultures have used the sun as a central focus to their beliefs. It was prominent in Ancient Egypt, and was the central symbol in the monotheistic beliefs of the Pharaoh Akhenaten. When used in conjunction with ancestral healing it can be applied in all cases where there is strong negative emotion.

## Cross

Best known are the Christian cross with its extended bottom limb, and the equal-armed cross. The Christian cross is connected with the development of Christianity and the

quality of self-sacrifice. Some people today find this particular form a restrictive symbol because of some of its associations. But those ancestors with Christian beliefs will often respond to the Christian cross, particularly when used in conjunction with forgiveness. In its equal-armed form the cross represents the balance of the four elements — earth, air, fire and water — within the physical material world. Jung appreciated the element's symbolic connection with aspects within our psyche and classified them in four categories: sensation, thinking, intuition and feeling.

## Cross within a circle/Celtic cross

This is an excellent symbol of balance, integration and protection. Circles have always been associated with the spirit. Combining the cross and the circle represents the link between the physical and spiritual side of our nature. It can therefore be used in all cases where this quality of integration is required. You can use it to balance chakric energies and also as a general symbol to surround an ancestor at the end of a healing session. (The chakras, traditionally seven in number, are energy centres located along the front of the body. The concept originated within the Vedic traditions and has now become generally accepted in healing, acupuncture, kinesiology and metaphysical belief systems.) The cross within a circle can have a very powerful protective quality if placed over areas of vulnerability or sensitivity in ourselves or others. Another form of this symbol is the Celtic cross. Where ancestors are concerned either of these symbols can be used where general balance is required.

## Chalice

A symbol of renewal and replenishment, the chalice can help link with the sensitive, feminine aspect of your being and carries a very gentle quality. It is the symbol of the Grail knights and as such is a most potent link with all spiritual seeking for inner wisdom. You can use it as a general healing symbol as well as one to provide you or your ancestors with a source of spiritual nourishment. Call upon it whenever you are feeling depleted in energy or low in spirits. Drinking a symbolic communion cup with your ancestors will allow their spiritual energy to connect to you.

## Caduceus

The Caduceus is symbol of Hermes, one of the principal healing gods of the Greek pantheon, the caduceus has been adopted by the modern medical profession. It represents the balance of energies as they move through the different layers within our being. Curiously, although it is a very ancient symbol it is very close to the shape of the DNA double helix molecule, which is the basic molecule of life. It can be used in all cases where balance is required, and specifically in balancing the masculine (yang) and feminine (yin) sides of our nature. The word 'hermaphrodite', which at a spiritual level represents the complete integration of the masculine and feminine principles within us, is derived from Hermes and Aphrodite, the goddess of love. You can use the caduceus in all cases where two opposing energies need to be united. It can also be used directly on the DNA to balance genetic disorders.

## Six-pointed star

This symbol too carries a powerful connection with the love energy. Six was considered the number of perfect harmony by Pythagoras and his followers. It also links with the quality of inner wisdom and can provide a gateway to other dimensions within our inner world. The Star of David, with its two interlocking triangles, is a version of this symbol. Use the six-pointed star in all cases where harmony with the ancestors is sought.

### Lotus

This symbol expresses the peace and serenity seen on the face of the Buddha. It is associated with meditation and inner seeking, strengthening the link between the physical body and the spiritual self. It is an excellent symbol to use with the ancestors when a feeling of peace and calmness is required.

### Working with symbols

You can either place the imagined symbol over your own head or draw upon its energy, or you can project the symbol directly to the patient. For example, if you wished to attract a feeling of inner peace you could visualize a lotus over your head and feel that energy flowing through you; alternatively you could place the lotus above the ancestor's head to bring forward that same feeling.

I use the symbols in both ways. Broadly speaking, I work with the major archetypal symbols such as the sun, Christ or particular gods or goddesses by sensing that I am linking to their energy and allowing it to flow through me. Specific symbols such as the caduceus I use directly upon the patient. For example, if I sense an imbalance between the masculine and feminine sides of an individual's nature I might superimpose the caduceus upon them and hold that symbol in my mind for as long as it felt appropriate.

Symbols, like colours, can be seen as an adjunct to healing skills. It is not necessary to use them to help your ancestors, but they can extend the range of perception and quality of energy that can be directed. The exercise below gives an example of their use in healing.

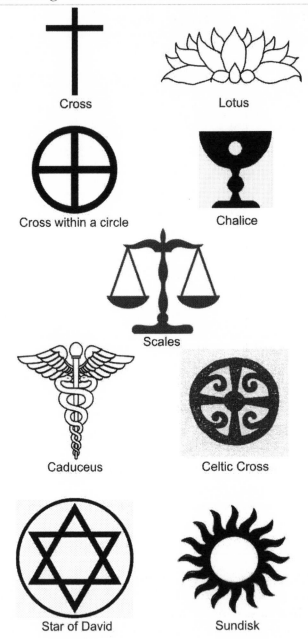

Cross

Lotus

Cross within a circle

Chalice

Scales

Caduceus

Celtic Cross

Star of David

Sundisk

## SYMBOL EXERCISE

### *Approximately 15 minutes*

**Aim:** *to extend your range of perception and quality of energy through the use of symbols*

- Sit comfortably as described for the exercise on p.148 and attune within by meditating quietly. Think of one of the symbols indicated above.
- First imagine that symbol over the top of your head. Draw the energy from the symbol into yourself and sense what you feel and experience.
- Now place the symbol under your feet and feel that you are drawing the energy up your body until you are completely surrounded by it. How do the feeling and sensation differ from those that you experienced in the first part of the exercise?
- Next place the symbol over the area of your heart and feel that you are linking your heart to the symbol. Again, how does this feel and what do you sense?
- Finally send out a thought of love through the symbol to a member of your family or one of your ancestors, and see what you experience.
- Gently bring yourself back to full waking reality and open your eyes.
- Write down what you experienced.

# Interpreting symbols

This is a huge subject, and whole books have been devoted to just one group of symbols. It is rather like learning a new language but one that, if mastered, can provide wonderfully fruitful insights into all sorts of situations. Into this category also come all the symbolic messages we receive in our dream world. An encyclopaedia of symbols can make the journey of interpretation very much easier and is strongly recommended. A number of good reference books are listed on pp. 200-204.

## Balancing opposites

Another important task is balancing opposites within the family tree. In Chinese philosophy, when energy reaches an extreme it will automatically reverse into its opposite: yin becomes yang, and vice versa. This principle was also perceived by the Greek philosopher Heraclitus, who called it enantiodromia. Jung and other family therapists have been aware of this dynamic both within individuals and within family groups. To achieve balance opposites must be present, but in order to experience it we need to move within a polarity. This is most pronounced in our gender for, in this life at least, you will be either a man or a woman. Generally, within our lifespan we move from one polarity to another quite freely, in the same way that we use each leg to walk. However, family dynamics may dictate that when one dynamic is powerfully present then its opposite will also be found within the family. Examples of this have already been given (see p.85) and can manifest, for instance, as the alcoholic of one generation being balanced by the teetotaller of the next.

Go back to your ancestors' chart and look at those associations that you put down from the different Degree listings (see pp.103-105). Note on a separate sheet of paper what you have uncovered. Let us say, for example, that you had one ancestor who was illegitimate, another who was convicted for theft, another who suffered from depression and one who frequently lost his temper. Think about this listing and try to determine what the opposite of each of these qualities might be. My suggestions would be as follows:

| **Quality** | **Opposite** |
|---|---|
| illegitimacy (sexual freedom or irresponsibility) | sexual inhibition or responsibility |
| theft or the tendency to steal from others | honesty and regard for others property |
| anger | never loses temper |

You might come up with other ideas, which is perfectly acceptable.

Now consider how both the primary quality and its opposite manifest in you. If you have a strong emotive reaction to one or any of these dynamics as they manifest within your own ancestors, believing that they could not possibly be part of you, then think again — they almost certainly are.

Next look for the ancestor who to you seems to carry the opposite of this quality. This may be found within the extended family, such as an uncle or aunt. If you are unsure or have no factual information to go on, use one of the intuitive systems given earlier (see Chapter 7).

The way to balance these energies within yourself is by acknowledging that both aspects of the polarity are present within your psyche. As soon as you reject one element you create imbalance within yourself, and that energy *has* to be carried by another. This will always be someone who is energetically linked to you, which will probably be a member of your family.

To balance these energies within your ancestral family, carry out the following exercise.

### POLARITY BALANCING EXERCISE
### *Approximately 10-15 minutes*

***Aim:*** *to balance the polarities within your own family*

- Choose one element that you wish to focus upon within your family. Let us suppose, for this example, that you have selected the quality of anger (it could equally be poverty, greed, abandonment and so on).
- Carry out the first two stages of the Healing exercise (see p.148), making sure that you connect to your inner light and H-S.

- Think of the particular ancestor who carries the quality of anger, and visualize them sitting in front of you.
- Next think of the ancestor who carries the opposite quality (patience, calm, passivity). If you do not know which ancestor that might be, imagine someone who could represent this and see them seated next to the original ancestor.
- Imagine that each ancestor is surrounded by their polarized qualities. To make this more real, you could associate a colour with each quality. Let us assume red is associated with anger and blue with the non-expression of anger. The first ancestor would then be surrounded by a red colour and the second by blue.
- Next visualize each colour being transmitted between the ancestors, so that the two colours merge together.
- Imagine the symbol of the scales in front of them, and hold this image in your mind until the scales seem balanced.
- Finally see the energy from these two ancestors flowing down the family tree in a balanced way to yourself, so that these energies are integrated properly with you.
- Thank both ancestors for their help and offer them into the light.
- Bring yourself back to full waking consciousness.

This exercise can be applied in all cases where a polarization of energy has taken place. You can also apply it if you consider that you are lacking in any particular quality. If, for instance, you feel unable to stand up for yourself, you could think of an ancestor who stood strong in their own space, as well as one who was weak. Link and balance their energies, using the exercise above, and feel connected to both polarities within yourself. In this way you will be linking with two ancestors to form a powerful triangular dynamic. Balance in this case would mean that you would know when to stand firm and when to retreat; both expressions are important in human relationships.

# Cleansing Ancestral Influences

It should be remembered that there are three primary driving forces that make us who and what we are. There is the influence from our upbringing, the influence from our ancestors and the influence from our spirit. Whilst with most people there is a broad balance in how these three sets of patternings work through us during our lives the most important is the influence that comes down to us from our spirit via the 'Higher-Self' (H-S). This part has the power to transform, transmute or overlay the other two elements. This is why the H-S can play such a significant role in healing traumas that stem from our childhood. In a similar way it can be used to heal and cleanse any distorted influence from our forebears. The following exercise shows how this can be done.

### TRANSMUTING ANCESTRAL INFLUENCES

*Approximate time 10 minutes*

**Aim:** *to cleanse any negative ancestral influences from the psyche*

- Close your eyes and carry out the body awareness exercise before linking to your H-S.
- Request your H-S to scan through your physical body and energetic body to highlight for you whether there is any negative genetic pattern that you are carrying within and to highlight this pattern as a colour.
- When you first do this exercise you will, almost certainly, see a colour in your imagination.
- Next call on your H-S to create a golden sieve and imagine that you are bringing this down from your H-S through the top of your head and through the whole of your physical body, catching within it

any residue of the colour that you perceived as being part of your ancestral influence.

- When the sieve is under your feet gather its content together and disperse this either back into the sun for transformation or if you prefer into the fiery regions of the earth.

- Repeat the sieving exercise two more times making a total of three in all.

- Now ask your H-S to indicate to you the colour of your inner soul essence and again you will get a colour coming into your mind.

- Imagine, sense or see inwardly this colour in the centre of your being perhaps located close to your heart and then see its energy radiating out through your physical body with a request that the colour and essence of your soul energy fills those areas where the resonance of the ancestral/genetic energy had resided.

- When this is done request your H-S to close and seal any doors, openings or windows within your psyche where ancestral/genetic energy had resided.

- Thank your H-S and healing guides and bring yourself back to full waking consciousness.

This exercise needs to be carried out again a week later and to ask again from your H-S whether there are any ancestral/genetic influences held within you. You will probably still see or sense a colour so repeat the exercise listed above. Again wait a week and carry out a re-check. This time you might or might not sense any residue of an ancestral/genetic link and if not simply strengthen the spiritual energy core of yourself and see this flowing through all levels of your being. If there is still some residue of ancestral/genetic influence remaining after this third clearing wait a month before repeating the process. You will ultimately fully cleanse and clear any ancestral/genetic influence from your psyche.

Based on this information one might wonder why there is any need to work to cleanse the ancestral influences, when these can simply be transmuted within oneself. It should be remembered that we are part of a family unit and many of us will have children or nephews and nieces and that they too can be influenced by any traumas held within the ancestral collective. To help clear and cleanse these influences is providing a service for the entire family.

# CHAPTER 10

# *Ancestral Dwellings*

Another important aspect of healing the past, which often requires attention, relates to places and in particular to family dwellings. Places and buildings hold patterns of energy derived from people who have lived in them. These patterns can be repeated, and re-emphasized, by whoever subsequently resides there. In this case, instead of one's own ancestors it is the ancestral inhabitants of the place who set up the pattern of influence. This is why houses acquire their own unique atmospheres. In the same way that it is important to feel a harmony of energy coming from your forebears, it is important to ensure that the energy of your home is in harmony with yourself.

In China the ancient art of balancing and harmonizing the energy of the home is known as Feng Shui, which literally means wind and water. These two elements symbolically represented the way in which subtle energy, known as Ch'i, flowed within a property. One Feng Shui master said that on one occasion he had rushed to acquire a property because the previous occupants had all started up very successful businesses before moving to new homes. As this was what he wished to do himself, it was important to make use of the beneficial energy of that place.

In recent years there has been a growing interest in the West in the ideas of Feng Shui and what individuals can do to improve the energies of their own homes — another aspect of the way in which energies from the past can influence our lives.

# The natural energy of places

Places have both a natural energy and an energy which has been created by human activity. In its beneficial form the first category includes the natural surroundings of the home, its proximity to trees, rocks, water, wind and sunshine, and that elusive factor that gives a place its special feel. In their more destructive form these same elements do not blend easily together: the place may be too damp, too exposed or infused by radon gas. Some people also suggest that there are other subtle distortions such as underground streams, geopathic stress and the like.

Human activity too can take two forms. The first involves all the emotional, psychological and spiritual activity that has taken place in the property, and the second the way that electromagnetic circuits, power cables and television sets influence the home environment.

Each of these areas can be tackled to improve the ambient energies of your home. Natural forces are the least amenable to change, although the Ancient Chinese would spend considerable time seeking to perfect the environment around their property. What can be more readily changed is the inherent ancestral energy patterns that have been generated by human activity. It is these energies that predominantly affect the lifestyle of people living within the home and become established as its ancestral energy matrix.

# Ancestral patterns in houses

The ancestral energies of homes are based on human activities that took place on that site before the property was built and on what has been generated within the property itself.

Considering the length of time that people have lived in Britain, and its density of population, it is unlikely today that you would find a site completely free from human involvement. With other places in the world you might be more fortunate. Any human activity will leave traces of energy at the place where that event occurred. Incidents such as ploughing a field or a discussion between two people do not have any lasting impact, but if a battle is fought on a site or a murder committed it will leave an imprint which will adversely affect those who subsequently come to that place.

In one property where I was asked to help there was extensive poltergeist activity. It was a modern house built on the site of a demolished Italian-style villa. The psychic phenomena had become so bad, with objects being thrown around the house, so that the owner had sought the help of the local priest who carried out an exorcism. Some improvement was noticed, but then a neighbour whose house backed on to the property started to suffer similar problems. It would seem that the exorcism had only shifted the problem into an adjoining house. After 'tuning in' to this property with one of my healing groups, we realized that the previous occupier of the villa, in his spirit form, was still around and, not appreciating that he was dead, was firmly convinced that people were trying to invade his home. Quite naturally he objected most strongly and was doing what he could to eject them. He was given healing and lifted from his 'earthbound' state so that he no longer bothered the living. Since carrying out that healing, no further disturbances have been reported.

Some friends living on the outskirts of London had been suffering a series of aggravating health problems. When I spent the night in their house I was very conscious of a disturbed energy that appeared to flow diagonally through the property. I asked a dowser to check this out, without telling him of my own findings, and he confirmed that he had felt a 'black' or disturbed energy line precisely where I had sensed it. In 'tuning in' to the energy of this line I felt that it went back to the time of the plague. It seemed that this had been a track-way used for carrying away plague-ridden bodies to be buried. A great deal of fear and suffering was still locked into the track. When I told my friend about all this he commented that his homeopath, without any logical reason, had recently given him an antidote to bubonic plague. This seemed an extraordinary coincidence. After healing and cleansing were carried out on the trackway there was a great improvement in its energies and the health of the family.

This is why the energies of brand-new homes can still sometimes feel very disturbed: they will have been built on sites that still carry such energies from the past. This situation can always be corrected, so a disturbed energy in itself need not necessarily put you off buying a house that is in other respects right for you. However, in the meantime you might find disturbing things happening.

Even if the site of your home is all right you will still be influenced by the various individuals who have lived there before you. These influences may only be very slight, but they will be there none the less. The good news is that, just as you can change the energies that you receive from your direct ancestors, so you can change the energies from the previous owners of your home. Before looking at this in more detail, here are a few words of general advice when buying a home.

Wherever possible, check out the previous use of the property. If it has been used in the past as some form of mental institution, you should be very wary. A good criterion is to ask yourself whether you would like to be in the company of the present or previous occupants for any length of time. If the answer is yes, it is quite likely that the atmosphere of the property will be suitable for you. But sometimes this check is not possible, or there may be other very good reasons why you need to buy that particular house or flat. A number of years ago I moved into a house that seemed very right to acquire, but it had a dreadful atmosphere. Fortunately I was in a position to do something about it and there was an immediate improvement in its feeling.

## Why do homes acquire atmospheres?

The easiest way to understand the influence of properties is to imagine each house as a computer that takes in all the data from the activities of its occupants. This computer also broadcasts back what has been fed into it, so that there is a two-way process going on all the time. Most people are completely unaware of this computer on a conscious level and think that by changing the decorations they can improve or alter the property to their own liking. Unfortunately this is not always so. The house computer will go on broadcasting its energies until the program is changed. If those energies have been particularly strong, it will start to nudge the new occupants into repeating the patterns laid down on the computer. It can have the effect of a subtle form of brainwashing, making the new people act in the same way as the previous occupants.

A married couple came to seek my help because they were suffering a breakdown in their relationship. They had inadvertently discovered that the marriages of the three previous owners of their home had split up, and they wondered whether the house was having any influence upon them. Sure enough, in 'tuning in' to the energy of the property I became aware of a particularly virulent aggressive energy from one of the previous owners. As soon as the 'house computer' had been accessed and the program changed the couple experienced a radical improvement in their relationship.

## Healing your home

It lies within most people's ability to improve or change the energy of their own home; however, I must issue a few words of warning. Just as the physical side of your house can sometimes reveal problems that require an expert, such as dry rot, you might need specialist help for this energetic level of healing. I would certainly recommend this level of assistance if you suspect the involvement of a spirit or ghost. Such souls are sometimes referred to 'earthbound' spirits. The vast majority of work that I undertake at this level is done from afar; as in healing people, a visit is not always necessary.

Ghosts are the spirits of those who have died but, for whatever reason, have not made the transition to the next plane. They remain stuck, usually through fear, to the place they knew best, which is their home. There are many reasons why the correct transition is not made. In some cases a violent death can tie a spirit to a place; in others the terror of thinking that they will go to hell for their misdeeds, however slight, will lock them in. I have also come across spirits in a comatose state who had died firmly believing that there was no such thing as an afterlife. Their conviction was so strong that it over-rode what would have been their normal transition. In other cases the spirit has not realized that it has died and continues to live out its previous existence. The man from the villa (see p.162) was an example of this type of phenomenon. In all these cases, by gently awakening these souls to their true position and then firmly helping them on their journey, a complete change is brought about. Difficulties in this type of healing only occur when the soul in question does not wish to move on. If not tackled correctly, there can be a psychic backlash which is most unpleasant.

## Earthbound Ancestors

Occasionally you may suspect that one of your own ancestors has become trapped or 'earthbound' and this was certainly the case within my own family tree. My father's mother, born in the latter part of the 19th century became pregnant before being married. The father was considered unsuitable by my great-grandfather and eventually my father was put up for adoption. My grandmother was now considered to be mentally unstable and the most appropriate treatment was for her to be put into a mental home, where she resided for nearly fifty years. I have never been able to discover the name of my grandfather, although I felt that he was bereft in leaving my grandmother and eventually died in the First World War. My grandmother died in the hospital where she had lived most of her life in 1963 but sadly she too was locked into the relationship and love that had been deprived from her. When I connected to her energetically I felt that she was still wandering around the hospital ward, with some part of her still looking for her lover. Through the power of higher consciousness I was able to connect with both my grandfather and my grandmother and to bring them both together again. The power of this experience was immense and the feeling of joy overwhelming. They were both then ready to move into the 'light' of the spirit world. What was most interesting from this experience was a radical change in attitude within my father, despite being in his eighties, although he had not been consciously aware of what I had done.

If you feel very confident about this type of release work then by all means carry this out for yourself. Otherwise I would suggest working it through with a therapist who specialises in this type of work.

## Resetting the house atmosphere

The exercise described below involves no more than clearing and resetting an atmosphere within a room, house or building — it does not involve the release of any earth-bound spirits. If you are working on your own home, and feel confident that there is no difficult energy around, by all means work on your own. Complete one room first before moving on to other areas of the property. First decide the method that you are going to use. Second, determine what is to be put in the place of the undesired atmosphere. There is a saying that 'nature abhors a vacuum'. If you take something out, you must put something back.

## Energetic cleansers

The most appropriate cleansers stem from the principles behind the elemental forces of fire and water, which are the two main cleansing agents of nature. In other words, imagine that you are either washing a room out with water, or burning up any disharmonious energy with fire. Some people work with air, visualizing a strong wind blowing the incumbent energy out of the house into the cosmos. This is fine at one level, but whilst it removes it from your own space you can end up dumping it on someone else.

The symbol I use most of the time is a flaming sword. I imagine I am holding the sword in my hand and then in my mind sweep through every part of the space cleansing the whole atmosphere, sending what is left out through the roof into the cosmos. If I choose to work with water, I would imagine a fine shower of rain falling through the room, washing away any impurities and taking the residue deep into the earth to be recycled.

Having carried out the clearing work, something needs to be put back. My recommendation would be to use one of the symbols or colours given in Chapter 9. As an alternative you could use the symbol of a flower, such as a rose of whichever colour or type that feels appropriate. You will need to draw on the energy behind the chosen symbol in exactly the same way that you do when giving healing, and sense that it is filling the whole of the cleared space. These energies are very tangible. On one occasion after I had cleared a property in France, the owner was convinced that I had sprinkled a lot of rosewater around the place for she could smell it strongly for several days afterwards. The only roses that had been used were the ones that had been planted at an imaginary level in the property. She was very surprised to find that we had not used any rosewater at all. I normally plant the symbol in the middle of the room and imagine its essence filling the whole space, either as a colour or just as a feeling.

Healing the energies of places in this way can bring a dramatic change of feeling, particularly if energies have built up over long periods of time. It is as though the house or room has been given a spring clean after years of neglect, though on an energetic rather than a physical level.

EXERCISE FOR CLEANSING AND SETTING AN
ATMOSPHERE IN A ROOM
*Approximately 10 minutes*

**Aim:** *to clear and reset the atmosphere of a room at a mental level*

- Adopt your normal healing/meditation postures.
- Close your eyes and attune within, connecting to your inner light. Ask also for help from the cosmos in what you are going to do and link to your H-S.

- Imagine that there is a strong bubble of light surrounding you and protecting you from any harmful energies.

- Now imagine that you have a flaming sword in your hand and sweep it around the room at least three times, cleansing everything in it. Finally see the smoke or residue flowing out through the roof into the cosmos.

- Next connect to the symbol and feel that you are drawing it down, planting the energy in the room. Sense that the feeling and quality of the symbol are filling every part of the space.

- Finally put a protection around the room, close down your energy and bring yourself back to full waking consciousness.

- When you have completed one room you can move on to the next.

For more details on this type of healing work, please read my book *Working With Earth Energies.*

When you have reset the energies of your house — symbolically changed its computer program — you will only occasionally need to check that everything is running smoothly. From experience, any imbalances that have been missed will usually show up very quickly and can be dealt with as they occur.

### Blessing your house

In conjunction with the cleansing exercise, when you move into a new home you could carry out a blessing ceremony to set up the right energies for what you want to achieve. If you have religious beliefs you could invite your local clergyman to perform the ceremony. A good alternative would be to invite some close friends who are sympathetic to your ideas and devise your own ceremony. Light a candle, burn some incense, say a prayer or do whatever you feel to be appropriate.

## Your home reflects you

Homes in dreams generally reflect an aspect of yourself. In guided imagery exercises, they are often seen as the part of ourselves that houses our inner nature. In its external form, like your ancestors it can exert a subtle influence on you. In thinking of your home in this light remember that you can change what surrounds you at this level. You do not have to be the victim of its energies, but can alter what is no longer appropriate for you.

# Epilogue

*'O Great Spirit, Great Spirit, my Grandfather — here at the centre of the world, where you took me when I was young and taught me; here, old, I stand, and the tree is withered, Grandfather, my Grandfather!*

*Again, and maybe the last time on this earth, I recall the great vision you sent me. It may be that some little root of the sacred tree still lives. Nourish it then, that it may leaf and bloom and fill with songbirds. Hear me, not for myself, but for my people; I am old. Hear me that they may once more go back into the sacred hoop and find the good red road, the shielding tree!'*

Thus spoke the famous Oglala Sioux medicine man Black Elk shortly before his death. His prayer for his own people carries a universal relevance. We each need to nourish and care for the tree that gave us birth — our family tree. It represents both the past and the future, woven together in a perfect symmetry. As we change the energies of the one, the other will surely follow suit.

This book has explored the different ways in which you can begin to connect to the rich heritage that your forebears bring. To some extent it focused on those aspects that need balancing within your family tree. Yet there is also the positive aspect of our ancestors' experiences. They too strove to understand, to preserve, to honour their beliefs and traditions; this is an enormous well of wisdom that we can draw upon in times of need and uncertainty. By unlocking the doors to our past, we open them to a future that can be unfettered by restrictive thinking. By loving your ancestors, for being who and what they were, you can ensure that the dynamic of their energies contributes something very positive into your life — something to be celebrated with great joy.

It is my hope that this book has inspired you to make the journey of connecting to and working with the energies of your own ancestors; that this will be as fruitful a journey for you as it has been for me in getting to know my own ancestors.

*'All that is needed is to reach the depths where transformation is effortless and most powerful. Our servants wait on us but they wait inside.'*

Deepak Chopra, *Journey into Healing*

# *Appendix*

Note: This section was originally written as an article. It is included here because of its relevance to the book. There are some duplications with the main text of the book and whilst it was considered that these could be removed or changed it was ultimately decided to leave them in as it helps the flow of ideas.

# Epigenetics, Soul Consciousness and Ancestral Healing

## Introduction

This paper explores the connection between epigenetics, soul consciousness and ancestral healing. Epigenetics is part of a revolutionary new science that is giving insights into how the DNA is modified to create the diversity of patterns that work through us. The word epigenetic is derived from the Greek word *'Epi',* which means above or around the genes (Spector, 2012) and implies an influence that affects how the genes operate within us. Soul-consciousness at root is the life force that distinguishes whether we are alive or dead. However, as we shall see from 'Near Death' studies, it also includes the notion of a consciousness that both operates through the medium of the physical body yet also would appear to be separate from it (Bray, 2013). Consideration will be given to how this primary aspect of the self links through to the physical body. Additionally it will be shown that by accessing our soul consciousness, higher mind, or God self, we can gain insights that allow for fundamental changes to take place within us. Ancestral healing is the methodology that can be used to clear patterns of influence that stem from the traumas of our forebears, such as divorce, deaths, illnesses and upbringing. These patterns predominantly stem from one's parents, grandparents and great-grandparents (Furlong, 1997). The concept here is that our ancestors are linked to us through genetic resonance and the lives that they led are still imprinted within the collective unconscious at an astral level. As part of our own self-healing process and to clear these patterns for future generations we need to access these levels of energy to heal and balance the dynamics that are contained there. We might like to consider this healing process as part of good internal house-keeping. The thesis will additionally examine the resonant links between epigenetics, soul consciousness and ancestral healing, showing how they might affect each other and concludes by suggesting that the connections between these fields highlights one of the potential bridging mechanisms between science and metaphysics.

# Epigenetics

**Background**

When Crick and Watson worked out in 1953 that the DNA was a double helix comprising four simple chemical bases, for which they obtained a Nobel prize, it was thought that the science was now well on the way to understanding the blueprint for life. This was further reinforced when scientists finally announced that the human genome had been sequenced in 2000. This feat was hailed as an amazing achievement and as US President Bill Clinton stated at the time: "*Today we are learning the language in which God created life*" (Carey, 2013). This optimism proved short-lived because science is now recognising that there is much greater complexity to this puzzle than they ever imagined. A number of awkward facts seemed to muddy the apparent perception of the genes as the sole repository of the patterns that make us who and what we are. As often happens these had been glossed over in the excitement of the first sequencing of the human genome but once this had been done and the realisation that instead of the 100,000 genes, human beings had around 23,000 only marginally more than the humble worm (Spector, 2012) it was clear that something else was required to explain the complexity of human development.

Since the start of the new millennium enormous strides have now been made into the field that would seem to explain, at least in part, the complexity of life. This new biology is called 'epigenetics', a term that was first coined by British biologist C.H. Waddington in 1942. Waddington followed this up with a now fully acclaimed concept referred to as 'Waddington's landscape', which he presented in his book 'The Strategy of the Genes' published in 1957. The model was an attempt to explain how a single cell, the fusion of one egg and one sperm, could develop to become one of the diverse two hundred or so different cells that make up the human body (Carey, 2013). Waddington's landscape portrayed a single cell like a round ball or marble rolling down a slope that then split into a number of different valleys, rather like the different tributaries at the delta of a river. It was thought that once the ball had reached the end of one or other of those tributaries that process could not then be reversed, or the ball rolled back up the slope to start again. Under normal conditions, this has to be the case because cells, once programmed, such as a liver cell need to know what their role is, within the scheme of our lives. However it is now known that this is not always true and that if thrust hard enough a fully developed cell can be reversed back to its original poly-potential state (Carey, 2013). Additionally DNA is now viewed rather differently than the pre-determined patterning that was originally conceived. An analogy might be to view our genome like the script of a play. It is a fixed script, yet one that can always be, modified or adapted depending upon the whims of the director. This is why no two performances of a play are ever identical; variations always occur (Carey, 2013). Epigenetics is now considered to include anything other than DNA for the heritable development of complex organisms (Holiday, 1990). Additionally the phenomenal developments in biology and chemistry have meant that we now have some tools to study how these changes take place, so that another level of epigenetics, includes the study of those mechanisms that produce the changes that we can observe (Carey, 2013)

## Recent Discoveries

Towards the end of the Second World War a starvation programme was inflicted on the Dutch population by the Nazi regime, during the exceptionally cold winter of 1944-45. In all some 20,000 individual perished but from this disaster an interesting study emerged. Because of excellent record keeping the lives of those children conceived just before or during this starvation period were then able to be monitored for the remainder of their lives. What was discovered was surprising in that those that had been conceived whilst food was readily available but then the mothers had been forced into starvation were all born small and below weight. Surprisingly they then continued to be below weight for the remainder of their lives, despite having access to plenty of food. Those conceived during the famine and then born after food was available were all obese and this obesity then continued on throughout their lives. This latter group was also much less healthy generally than those of the first group. Additionally it has now been discovered that the children of these original children, or the grandchildren of the original mothers contain similar characteristics. These environmental patterns had effectively been passed on to the grandchildren (Carey, 2013). This was a startling discovery because the whole edifice of Darwin's theory is based on the premise the gene mutations are random and are only very slowly absorbed into a population over many generations (Darwin, 1859). The Dutch study showed this not to be the whole story. Since then studies in mice have duplicated the result of the Dutch research and it is now known that environmental changes in foetal development can be passed on to subsequent generations (Carey, 2013).

Prior to Darwin's theory another researcher called Jean-Bapiste Lamarck had suggested in his most famous work 'Philosophie Zoologique', published at the beginning of the

19th century that acquired characteristics can be transmitted from one generation to the next and that this is the driver of evolution. For many years after Darwin's theories became established the heresy of Lamarck's ideas were considered with ridicule (Carey, 2013). Whilst the broad thrust of Darwinian theory is right, in some cases patterns are clearly passed on from one generation to the next. How this might work out in the long term is not yet understood (Carey, 2013).

The biology and chemical reactions that give rise to these epigenetic effects are now being closely studied and some discoveries have been made showing how the genes can be turned off and on in response to specific stimuli. It is now thought that cancer could be an example of an epigenetic mutation, where the switching mechanisms have gone wrong and research is now starting to target these processes (Carey, 2013). They way these patterns work through us has also been highlighted from numerous twin studies, which will now be discussed.

## Twin Studies

Twins born from the same sperm/egg are commonly known as identical twins, although the correct name is monozygotic (MZ). These twins share 100 per cent the same genes, in other words an analysis of their DNA would be the same in both cases. Sets of monozygotic twins provide a rich source of potential information because it becomes possible to determine the degree of heritability of any one physical factor, such as the colour of the eyes or their height, when compared with fraternal or non-identical twins (Spector, 2012). Over the years millions of separate twin studies have been carried out to try to assess the role of the environment against heritability, which centres in the classic nature/nurture debate. The tendency has been for the pendulum to swing between these two polarities over the space of many years. What the twin studies show is that whilst DNA patterns are established within an environmental setting, which affects the development of an individual, little is immutable and that most aspects of us have the potential for change (Spector, 2012).

Perhaps the first most obvious element is that even though carrying exactly the same DNA, the twins themselves always have individual characteristics; even in the case of Siamese twins. Two identical twins, Laleh and Ladan, were conjoined in the head area and grew to adulthood through twenty-three years. Despite having the same DNA and being exposed to the same environment, through virtue of their condition, they had very different personalities, which were fully analysed through different studies. Laden liked animals, whilst Laleh preferred computer games, which Laden could not stand. One was left-handed the other right and they both were studious, with Laden hoping to be a lawyer and Laleh a journalist. It was clear from the onset that Laden was the more extrovert and talkative of the two twins. Ultimately their quest of separate identity and life lead them to an operation where their two heads and the conjoined brain tissue would need to be divided in an operation (Spector, 2012). We might reflect on the courage of these two individuals whose desire for a separate life was so powerful that they were prepared to put their own lives at risk to achieve such a result. Sadly the operation when performed was not successful and both Laleh and Laden died on the operating table, without gaining consciousness, separated at least in death (Spector, 2012).

What this and many other monozygotic (MZ) twin studies show is the power of the individual personality within each twin. They are far from being clones of each other and each twin within a pair set will have their own unique personality traits, even though some of their mannerisms might be similar. These changes would appear to start very early on within foetal development (Carey, 2013) and this raises the question what might be the factor that leads to this individuation process, which as we have seen the case of Laleh and Ladan was so powerful that they were prepared to face death rather than continuing in their incapacitated state, despite being very good friends. Before looking at this question in some depth in the next section something needs to be said about the underlying patterns that make us who and what we are and the role that heredity might play in this arena. To do this we need to look again at identical twins, although in this case twins that have not been raised together but raised apart; twins that formed part of the famous Minnesota Twin study carried out by Professor Bouchard.

The story started in 1979 when Jim Lewis, then 39 years old, decided to track down his brother who had been living locally. They had been separated soon after birth and adopted into two different families. When they eventually met up again they discovered a series or remarkable coincidences that had run through their individual lives. Both called Jim, they had each been married to a woman called Linda and then divorcing her married a Betty. They had both named their eldest son James Alan Lewis and James Allen Springer, the only difference being in the spelling of the name Alan. They both had smoked Salem cigarettes and drank Miller Lite beer. They had similar IQs, liked maths and hated spelling and they both drove the same model and colour Chevrolet. These 'coincidences' were so notable that they eventually came to the attention of Professor Bouchard, who then initiated his twin study seeking out monozygotic twins who had been reared apart, with the intention of being able to assess the roles of both heredity and environment in gene expression. Twins reared apart would generally have very different environmental similarities showing that any congruence is likely to have a genetic element (Spector, 2012).

The discoveries from the Bouchard surveys showed that in some cases there was a remarkable level of congruence between monozygotic twins with in some cases correlations in dates when key events like marriages, diary keeping, illnesses and so on occurred synchronistically, suggesting that there are potential levels of patterning within us that can influence how we act, which seem to stem from our genetic inheritance. Nevertheless this degree of patterning did not occur within all twins, suggesting that individuals could break out of these underlying trends and act from their own perspective (Spector, 2012).

One aspect of the twin studies looked at the influence of heredity on personality types, dividing individuals into five main categories of *Extraversion, Neuroticism, Conscientiousness, Agreeableness* and *Openness.* The converse or negative aspects of these personality types were also considered. For example the negative aspect of *agreeableness* was *aggressive, unfriendly, quarrelsome, cold* and *vindictive* (Bouchard, 1994). From these studies it was shown that about 42% of our personality could be traced to a genetic influence (Bouchard, 1994). In consideration of all of these factors Bouchard suggests that:

> *"Current thinking holds that each individual picks and chooses from a range of stimuli largely on the basis of his or her genotype and creates a unique set of experiences - that is people help to create their own environments."*

(Bouchard, Science, Vol. 264, [1994] p.1701)

## Conclusion

Studies in epigenetics show that there are a wide range of influences that affect the development and life patterns of any person and whilst heredity elements are significant creating a tendency, within all monozygotic twins towards toward similarity, of equal importance are the differences. In the course of these studies a number of assumptions have needed to be overturned. The first is that the DNA or your genes are the essence of you, the blueprint code of your life. The concept of the 'selfish gene' of Richard Dawkins is simply a myth (Spector, 2012). Although genes are an important part of the pattern, they do not act alone and other factors have equal status.

The second assumption is that *'genes and heritable genetic destiny cannot be changed'* (Spector, 2012). We now know that except in rare circumstances this is not the case. If this were so each set of MZ twins would always express the same illnesses and they do not. For example, whilst Schizophrenic episodes occur in about 1 per cent of the population if one MZ twin becomes schizophrenic there is a 50 per cent chance that the other will contract the illness. If the genetic pattern was fully predetermined then the congruence should be a 100 per cent (Carey, 2013). The 50 per cent difference needs to be understood and explained.

The third assumption is that significant environmental events *"cannot plant a lifelong memory within your cells"* (Spector, 2012). It was believed that every time a cell divided the information that it contained was effectively wiped clean, rather like reformatting a computer disk. We now know that memories can be passed on to future cell patterning particularly where events have occurred in foetal development or the early stages of a child's life. The example of the Dutch famine children illustrates this effect (Spector, 2012).

The final assumption is that the experiences of your parents or grandparents, particularly in relationship to environmental influences cannot be passed on to you, as suggested by Lamarck's theories. The evidence is clear that such inheritance does indeed occur, although the precise way this works out through the individual is always subject to many different factors (Spector, 2012).

In the next section of this thesis we will explore one of those potential factors.

# Soul Consciousness

**Background**

The concept of the '*soul*' or life essence has ancient origins. To the early Greeks it was known as the 'psyche'; to the ancient Egyptians the 'Ba', symbolised by a bird with a human head. In all cultures up to the 19th century, the existence of this part of our make-up was an accepted fact. However with the development of scientific study and the exploration into mind, brain body links the dualistic concept that saw a separation between the soul/mind and the body was consigned to the dustbin and became part of scientific heresy. Even today, despite many advances in scientific awareness and evidence the majority of scientists cannot conceive consciousness as being separate from the body (Bray, 2012). This section will examine the evidence that undermines this rigid materialistic stance.

### Near Death Studies

In a seminal book published in 1975 entitled 'Life after Life' Doctor Raymond Moody first made known to the general public a phenomenon that is now called the 'Near Death Experience' or NDE for short (Moody, 1975). NDEs are associated with the near clinical death of an individual or where a person has apparently died for a short period of time. Modern medical intervention in treating heart attacks, strokes, accidents or close to death events has meant that some individuals have been revived from unconsciousness or coma, when the threshold of death would appear to have been crossed. During this state around 18 per cent of individuals experience an NDE (Sartori, 2014). This involves first feeling separated from their body and having a sense of being able to observe what is happening to them in the revival process. A smaller subset might then experience travelling through a tunnel of light, where they might meet deceased relatives or sometimes a great being of light, generally experiencing powerful feelings of peace and love at this stage. At some point they are told or encouraged to return back to their body and then perceive themselves being drawn back into the physical. Here is a typical example taken from a *Daily Mail* article in 1995 by Graham Turner. It recounts the experiences of a woman in her mid-forties who very nearly died from pneumonia. Passing from her body, she travelled down a tunnel of light and then found herself standing in a beautiful field. The story continues:

> *"On my right was a wooden bench, the sort that you see around playing fields. It hadn't got any arms on it. There sat my Grandpa Tuck who died eight years before. I went over and sat next to him.*

`Are you all right, girl?' he asked.

`Yes,' I replied, 'I'm fine.' He was as real to me as my daughter Angela. He was dressed as he used to be, old cloth cap, jacket and working overalls, as if he hadn't died at all. It's really weird looking back on it.

I told him I didn't want to go back. 'You've got to go, girl,' he said, 'for the sake of the kids.' I couldn't bear the thought and I wasn't worried about the kids either. I remember thinking that my husband was quite capable. I said: 'You will come back for me when my time comes, won't you?' and he said: 'Yes, I'll be back after four ... ' Then there was a kind of electric shock, and I came back in intensive care."

(Turner, cited in Furlong, 1997 p. 15)

From this account it is clear that the woman felt the conscious part herself to be in a very different place from where her body resided.

One of the normal challenges from those that cannot accept this separation of consciousness from the body is that this is simply due to oxygen deprivation and a trick of the brain. To counter this argument researcher Dr Elizabeth Kübler-Ross sought out blind people who had had a near death experience to discover what they might have experienced. Eventually she found some who had been blind for at least ten years and discovered that they were able to give detailed evidence of the type and colour of clothes that people were wearing at the time that the incident happened. As she so rightly states "blind people cannot do this." (Kübler-Ross, 2011, YouTube interview).

In an eight year study of 'near death' experiences Dr Penny Sartori became convinced that this was a genuine phenomenon (Sartori, 2014). She began her studies from the viewpoint of the sceptic as, at the time, she was an intensive care nurse with over seventeen years experience who had become interested in what happened when people died. She came to her new conclusions from extensive observation and study. One account that she cites of an individual called

Tom, who despite being in a coma for three hours was able to describe clearly the efforts to resuscitate him. When eventually he regained consciousness he felt a complete loss of the fear of death and more telling, his right hand, which had been frozen at birth into a claw like shape because of contracted tendons, suddenly flexed and opened out. As Sartori states there is no medical explanation as to how this could happen (Sartori, 2014).

Through her studies she has been able to show that all of the medical or physical explanations for NDE's do not hold much credibility and little scientific study has been carried out to support these contrary assertions. For example, she was able to extract blood from two patients who had an NDE and found that their oxygen levels were perfectly normal, ruling out the claim these experiences are due to oxygen deprivation (Sartori, 2014).

One of the most notable features of the majority of those that go through these experiences is the sense that this was a significant and often life-changing event that firstly removed all fear of death and secondly often brought with it some profound changes in personality, life-style and sometimes physical health, such as the account of Tom above. In February 2006, Anita Moorjani slipped into a coma, for what her husband and family thought was the last time. She had been suffering from advanced lymphoma, which had reached stage III, where the cancer had spread throughout her lymph system and none of her doctors thought she had long to live. During the various medical procedures to bring her back she was fully aware and conscious of what was taking place, although feeling no pain or attachment to her physical body. She then started to fully separate from her body and became aware of her father who had passed over several year before her. He then started to tell her about her life and the reasons why she had contracted cancer. The sense of love that emanated from him and other beings was immense; she knew that she had a choice as to whether to continue on into the spirit world or to return back to the physical. She began to become aware of the power within her own spirit, in a sense getting in touch with her true self. As she stated:

> *"As though to confirm my realisation, I became aware of both my father and Soni ( a close friend who had also died of cancer) communicating to me: Now that you know the truth of who you really are, go back and live your life fearlessly."*

(Moorjani, 2012 p. 76)

She returned back to her body and regained consciousness and then started a steady journey back to full health. In her particular case it took just a fortnight before tests showed that there was not a single trace of cancer now within her body. The soul essence part of her being had brought about a complete reversal of a disease at a speed that was considered impossible (Moorjani, 20012). Moorjani has since gone to write about her experiences to deliver the message of how to live our lives fearlessly.

In another amazing case singer song writer Pam Reynolds had a near death experience whilst undergoing brain surgery in 1991 that necessitated the complete shut-down of her brain and heart during a full hour operation to clear an aneurism at the base of her brain. During this period all brain activity was flat-lined, effectively showing that there should have been no conscious awareness at all. Yet nevertheless Pam initially saw what was going on during the first stages of the operation. She then felt herself travelling through a tunnel of light to meet individuals that she knew had already passed over. She felt herself standing in the breath of the light of God. She then returned back to her body and eventually with a little persuasion from her uncle she moved back into her physical self and then slowly started to regain consciousness, eventually leading to a full recovery. From the evidence she presented it seemed impossible for her to have been aware of any part of the operation, yet nevertheless this is what happened (Sabom, 1998). Sceptics naturally have claimed that these memories must have occurred either just before the operation began or after the end or perhaps the equipment was not good enough to record brain activity. As the online Skeptics Dictionary states:

> "At this point in our knowledge, to claim that NDEs provide strong evidence that the soul exists independently of the body, and that there is an afterlife awaiting that soul that just happens to coincide with the beliefs and wishes of the near-death experient seems premature."

(Caroll, 2014 see website: http://www.skepdic.com/nde.html )

It is clear from the above statement that the sceptic will always look for ways of trying to understand these experiences in rational, mechanistic terms and probably no amount of hard evidence will ever convince them otherwise. Their position might be considered somewhat akin to a particular stance taken in what is now known as Young's double slit light experiment, where light can be observed as either waves or particles depending upon the observer's viewpoint. By applying the rational mechanistic or classical mechanical view to observing light it is only possible to perceive light as discreet particles not as waves and yet the experiment shows that it is both. It is only when perceived through quantum mechanics that the paradox can be explained (See ChemEurope.com for a detailed explanation). It requires a mindset other than the mechanistic to accept or understand NDE's.

### Reincarnation and Past Lives

NDE's are but one element that gives credence to the existence of the soul. Another stems from the researches of hypnotherapists many of whom go on to discover deep traumas within clients that appear to stem from previous lives. By intervening and helping the client move through the trauma relief to a current medical condition is obtained. One such story recounted in Dr Denis Kelsey's book *Many Lifetimes* involved a friend that had come to stay with the Kelseys for a short visit during the winter season. At the end of the stay as a parting gift the Kelseys produced a pheasant for cooking, which had been killed a few days earlier. As soon as the guest saw the pheasant they fainted. It transpired that all their life they had an extreme terror of feathers classically known as Pteronophobia. After regaining consciousness and explaining the problem the guest agreed to a regression session where they felt they had been caught up in a Crusader battle and had been fatally wounded. The apparent normal process would have been for their comrades to finish them off after the battle but in this case the soldier was left and his final memory was of vultures starting to eat his body. Through suggestion the intensity of this memory was released and thereafter all fear of feathers dissolved. Clearly some deep emotional connection must have occurred in this instance between these two apparent lifetimes (Grant and Kelsey, 1969).

Isolated instances, such as this, on their own account for very little yet when added together represent a caucus of knowledge that is hard to refute. Another researcher Michael Newton took the process one stage further in his books *Journey of Souls*, *Destiny of Souls* and *Memories of the Afterlife*, where he developed a technique for helping people access into memories of between life states. These he considered helpful in allowing clients to gain insight into why they had chosen to be born into a particular life and how current life often reflected a pattern of previous incarnations (Newton, 1994). Like NDE's Newton's extensive client base showed a similarity of experience when accessing this between life state, suggesting the regressed patients were indeed accessing another level of consciousness. The information suggested both a post life review of a life just completed as well as a careful selection for a new life and the opportunities that it offered. The perception being that the particular body was carefully chosen and then programmed by the incoming soul (Newton, 1994). This could be an explanation for the differences perceived in MZ twins, for two distinct souls would inevitably create a different set of patterns despite the identical DNA.

Other researchers, such as Jungian analyst Roger Woolger author of *Other Lives, Other Selves* confirm the pattern of soul expression through different lives seeking to balance issues between one life and the next. The book cover states:

> *"Illustrated with hundreds of anecdotes and moving case histories, 'Other Lives, Other Selves' investigates the connection between past life illness and current life health – both emotional and physical. Some of the more common psychological issues which have responded to past life regression are insecurity, phobias, depression and sexual difficulties. Dr Woolger also examines reincarnation philosophy to shed light on the multiplicity of the human personality, the psychology of karma and both Buddhist and Hindu perspectives."*
> (Woolger, 1999 *Other Lives, Other Selves* book cover)

It is clear from these many experiences of his different clients and those that attended his courses that the conscious aspect of the self (Soul) programmes the psyche and the physical body with specific sets of patterning. One such being the frequency of wound injuries carried over from one life to the next, sometimes appearing a birth mark scarring (Woolger, 1999). Woolger was not the first to spot this type of physical patterning. Professor Ian Stevenson in his famous and very detailed study entitled *"Twenty Cases Suggestive of Reincarnation"* highlights a number of such cases where wounds have shown as birth skin defects in the current life (Stevenson, 1988). This is highly suggestive of some level of physical imprinting from an epigenetic source.

### Dissociative Identity Disorder

The final area worthy of consideration with respect to the imprinting of the physical from a psycho spiritual source relates to those individuals suffering from Dissociative Identity Disorder (DID), which was originally known as Multi-Personality Disorder. It is now thought that DID cases reflect a fragmentation of the psyche, where separate and clearly identified different personalities assume control from time to time. These parts are generally known as 'alters' and there is generally one executive part that retains some level of overall control. A most remarkable case of this illness is author Kim Noble whose book *"All of Me"* describes her experience of dealing with more than twenty different and distinct personalities that assume control of her body at different times (Noble, 2011). Most of these personalities have no recollection of each other thereby creating a lot of inner havoc within Noble's life. She has however managed to bring up a daughter, now aged sixteen and develop as an accomplished artist. As her daughter states, she immediately knows when one personality steps back and another takes over (Noble, 2011). Included in this mix of personalities are a number of women of different ages, a boy called Diabalus who only speaks Latin and French and Ken, a gay man trying to come to terms with society's treatment of homosexuality. Each has his or her own personality and health quirks that affect the body that is called Kim, (Noble, 2011). In other DID cases these changes can be extreme. In a scholarly article by James Chu, published in the Journal of Trauma and Dissociation he states:

> *"There is a long history of reports of psychophysiological differences between the alternate identities in DID. Case reports include markedly different handwritings, variable visual acuity, medications responses, allergies, plasma glucose levels in diabetic patients, heart rate, blood pressure readings, differential EEG patterns, neural network patterns on functional magnetic resonance imagery (FMRI), and differences in brain activation and regional blood flow using single positron emission computed tomography (SPECT), among others (Loewenstein&Putnam,2004, Putnam, 1984, 1991b; Sar, Unal, Kiziltan, Kundakci, & Ozturk,2001)"*
>
> (Chu, Journal of Trauma and Dissociation Vol. 6(4) 2005 p. 117-118)

In all of these cases the researchers and therapists do not make any judgement on the origin of the 'alters' or personalities. In some ways they do not seem too different from the sub-personalities experienced in psychotherapy. However they may be separate souls or soul fragments that are able to gain momentary or partial control of the body for a specific period of time. During these phases the 'alters' can exhibit different physiological conditions such as the allergic reaction to different substances, where the same body will have a different reaction depending on which 'alter' is dominant (Chu, 2005). This shows that consciousness has a direct influence, sometimes startling so, on the epigenetic patterning of the body, suggesting that some of these patterns must stem directly from the personality that is then dominant.

## Conclusion

There is substantial evidence for the existence of an aspect of consciousness that can survive the death of the physical body. For want of a better word we can call this part the soul. It is clear from the above evidence that this aspect of our being has the potential to directly affect the epigenetic patterns that make us who and what we are. What is also apparent is that these patterns are not fixed and immutable but can be changed with remarkable speed when modified. The change from advanced lymphoma, with golf ball sized tumours, to a normal healthy body in the space of two weeks as in the case of Moorjani, shows just how rapid these changes can be (Moorjani, 2011). The almost instantaneous allergic switching that occurs in DID cases is another example. What is apparent is that our physical body, although the product of ancestral and environmental patterning, is also under our control at a psycho-spiritual and mental level. We have the ability to change and modify the expression of our genetic inheritance. In the next section we will explore how this might be done.

# Ancestral Healing

## Background

The concept of ancestral patterns affecting a current life has ancient origins. In the Bible we read:

> *You shall not bow down to them or worship them; for I, the LORD your God, am a jealous God, punishing the children for the sin of the parents to the third and fourth generation of those who hate me.*
> Exodus 20:5

and

> *As He passed by, He saw a man blind from birth. And His disciples asked Him, "Rabbi, who sinned, this man or his parents, that he would be born blind?"*
> John 9:2

From the above statements it is clear that the concept of some form of ancestral patterning (the sins of the fathers) was an accepted part of Jewish cultural belief.

It is known that many archaic cultures, such as the Ancient Egyptian, incorporated ancestor worship, within their belief systems (Furlong, 1997) and even today one of the main religions of Japan, Shintoism is based on a form of ancestor worship. In his book *Karma and Reincarnation* Dr Hiroshi Motoyama, head priest of the Shinto Tamamitsu sect of Japan, makes this profound statement:

> *"The parent/child connection manifests as one link in a long chain of ancestral karma that stretches back through time. Your link to your family allows you to be born into that specific line — it is a link that needs to be understood and respected. In this modern scientific age it is very difficult for people to accept the fact that they are responsible to their ancestors, that they are actually liable for the actions of their ancestors if the resulting karma has not yet been dissolved. Many find it absurd to think that the actions of an unknown ancestor could possibly have anything to do with what is happening to them today. But time and time again when*

*investigating someone's karma, I find problems that stretch back generations. Their spirit is not just an individual entity, it is also part of the family spirit that births and nurtures it."*
(Motoyama, 1998 p. 52)

In many cultures it was considered that the ancestral spirits were a fixed commodity on the basis that their behavioural patterns expressed during their lifetimes would go on being replicated in the same way in the afterlife. The benign ancestor could be approached easily but the aggressive ancestor needed to be treated warily (Furlong, 1997). We now know that these ancestral patterns are not fixed and immutable but can be healed and changed. The next section of this thesis will explore the methods that can be used (Furlong, 1997).

As the Bible states it is generally the patterns that stem from the first three generations that are the most important; in other words your parents, grandparents and great grandparents, making fourteen ancestors in total. It is clear that the further back one travels in time the more diluted becomes any specific ancestral pattern, although it is true to say that similarities of specific traumas can get passed on from one generation to the next (Furlong, 1997). This is perhaps why Motoyama suggests problems that can stretch back generations. It is possible using a little maths to understand something of the size of your ancestry. Go back ten generations, or approximately 300 years and you will have a total of over a thousand ancestors in that ancestral line making a grand total of more than two thousand ancestors in all. Travel further back to thirty generations and the number grows to a staggering one billion, with a combined total of more than two billion ancestors. A generation or two more and the number would be in excess of the current world population. Naturally there was not that number of people on the planet at the time, which shows that we are all closely related. In his seminal book *The Seven Daughters of Eve*, Professor Brian Sykes has been able to demonstrate, using mitochondrial DNA analysis, that the majority of the European population was descended from just seven women (Sykes, 2001).

## Changing DNA Patterning

In the mid-fifties a young boy with a severe skin problem was diagnosed as having a serious outbreak of warts. His doctor heard that hypnotism sometimes worked in these cases and referred him to Dr Albert Mason, a clinical hypnotist at the Queen Victoria Hospital in East Grinstead. The boy proved to be an excellent subject, and through hypnotic suggestion his condition began to clear up. In the meantime, just to be sure that the original diagnosis was correct, a sample of skin tissue was analysed. The results revealed that the boy was suffering not from warts, which are caused by a virus, but from congenital Ichthyosis or fishskin disease, a hereditary condition for which there was no known cure (Mason, 1952).

In theory it was impossible for the boy to have made any recovery just through the suggestions of the hypnotist; yet the results were there for all to see. Certainly the hypnotist thought at first that he was dealing with warts and therefore believed strongly in the possibility of a cure. Over the next four years a 60-70 per cent permanent improvement was achieved (Mason, 1952). This reinforces the perception that it is possible, under the right circumstances, for the messages coming from our genetic code to be modified by the mind, particularly where access is made through to the sub-conscious self via hypnotic suggestion.

A review of the literature of the medical use of hypnosis shows its extensive use in a wide area of health treatments that includes physical conditions as well as psycho-somatic, emotional and mental problems (Appel, 2003).

## Healing and Releasing Ancestral Patterns

One of the first books to tackle the concept of healing ancestral patterning was written by Dr Kenneth McAll in 1986. The book was entitled 'Healing the Family Tree'. McAll was a consultant psychiatrist and an Associate Member of the

Royal College of Psychiatrists, who had spent part of his early life in China. He had a deep and powerful connection to Christianity and to Christ consciousness, where he felt Jesus was actually communicating directly to him (McAll, 1986).

One of the stories he recounted in his book was of a woman who came to see him because she had developed a disturbing phobia about drowning. The fear had started when she was with her young children on a shallow boating lake and, in messing about, they succeeded in tipping the boat over. Because the lake was not deep there was little danger but from that moment an irrational fear of drowning pervaded the woman's mind. After seeing Dr McAll the woman did some research into her family tree and discovered that an uncle of hers had drowned when the Titanic sank in 1912 (McAll, 1986).

The approach taken by McAll was different from what might have been expected. He arranged for a Christian memorial service to be held in which his patient played an active part. As soon as the service was completed the woman felt the fear leave her and thereafter was completely free of the phobia (McAll, 1986). We might surmise that the spirit of her ancestor, or perhaps just the energy pattern that stemmed from him, was the cause of the problem; perhaps at some level he was still stuck or 'earthbound'. It is also possible that the woman was the reincarnated spirit of the uncle. Whatever the source of origin by healing her ancestor she had effectively healed herself. In this particular case it was not even her direct forbear but reflected something the spirit of Motoyama's concept of being responsible to our ancestors and the requirement to clear family karma.

In another example a member of the clergy came to see McAll because his daughter had been sectioned under the Mental Health Act; the reason being that she felt an overwhelming urge to gouge out her children's eyes. This became so serious that the only approach seemed to have her hospitalised in a mental institution more than a hundred miles away. After some research into their family tree they discovered that an ancestor living in the Middle Ages had been connected to a castle where implements of torture were found for gouging out people's eyes. They did not know whether the ancestor was involved although they suspected this might be the case. McAll again arranged a Christian service of healing and forgiveness for the release of any karmic energy sending prayers to the ancestor for the release of his soul. After the end of the service, in which only the father was present, they checked back to find out how the daughter was. To their amazement the discovered that she now felt completely free from the compulsion and was able shortly afterwards to be re-united with her family and children. Even more compelling was the discovery that an aunt, who suffered from schizophrenia, although knowing nothing on what was going on, was also instantaneously healed (McAll, 1986).

These cases graphically demonstrate how patterns that stem from our ancestors can flow down into the family dynamic affecting different members in unique ways. By learning to heal these patterns we can consciously clear our family karma.

## Methods of Healing Family Patterns

Family therapy will often entail looking at past patterns as well as the current family dynamic. These tend to be specialist sessions picking up specific issues and problems that might be manifesting in different ways within a family. These therapeutic sessions are generally restricted to small select groups where specific issues have manifested. Yet we all have ancestors and there is a potential for all of us to be affected at different levels by some of their past traumas. As has been shown with studies in epigenetics, patterns from the past do get relayed on down to us all. Therefore the ideal situation would be to take steps to clear and release these patterns as part of helping the family karma, not only for us, but also for our children and our children's children.

The approach suggested here has been developed from a number of different sources over many years. Perhaps the best starting point is the book by Dr Tom Zinser entitled "*Soul Centred Healing: A Psychologist's Extraordinary Journey into the Realms of Sub-Personalities, Spirits and Past Lives*", which was published in 2011. Dr Zinser was a hypnotherapist who worked with trying to heal the emotional traumas of his clients by helping them directly connect with their sub-personalities or 'ego-states' and the patterns of energy that they held. The technique he used to access these sub-personalities was based on putting the clients into a light hypnotic trance and the use of ideo-motor signalling (Zinser, 2011). This process proved rather hit and miss until one of his secretaries mentioned that she had a spiritual guide who worked with her called Gerod and this guide wished to help Zinser in his therapeutic work. From that point on Zinser had regular sessions with the guide to try to get a better understanding of what was taking place and the steps he needed to take to get the client's back into full health and inner balance. Eventually he was able to hone this therapeutic approach to a number of simple steps (Zinser, 2011). Crucial to this process was the support and help derived from the client's own 'Higher-Self' (H-S). We might call this the client's Divine Self . In essence all inner work needs to come under the guidance and support of this part of the client's being because the H-S part has a full overview and knows what steps need to be taken to resolve any internal issues. Additionally it has the power to correct any problems once the lesson has been understood and learned (Zinser, 2011).

Interestingly the concept of an inner wise being or 'inner self helper' had been recognised in hypnotherapy and psychotherapy many years earlier by those working with the sub-personality parts of the self. The term Inner Self Helper (ISH) was first coined by psychologist Ralph Allison in his book *"Minds in Many Pieces: The Making of a Very Special Doctor."* Allison came to realise that there was a part of the psyche that seemed to have a handle on what was happening within some very disturbed clients and could be very helpful, providing it could be readily accessed through hypnotherapy (Allison, 1980). However it is not quite clear whether Allison perceived the ISH in the same light as Zinser came to view the 'Higher-Self'.

From my own perspective, being brought up in Christian Science and being a healer all of my life, I have had an awareness of working with specific levels of spiritual energy to support and help the client's that I work with. It was this healing work that led to the publication of my different books on healing. The concept of Christian Science is premised on a very simple idea namely God is perfect, we all have an aspect of God within us and all we need to do is recognise this state of inner perfection, the manifestation of the God principle, for us to be healed (Eddy,1875). This simple idea is very effective in many cases, although it does not work all of the time, or rather not all individuals can easily work with this concept.

My quest then has been to find ways and methods of healing, by connecting to this place of inner knowing, to help resolve the issues and problems that might impact upon us. Independent of Tom Zinser's work I had come to recognise something similar about helping the client to access their own 'H-S' to gain insight into what needs to be done to clear and resolve sometimes very difficult spiritual, psychological and mental issues. This methodology can be applied to all aspects of healing and is at root very simple. The technique will be described here being directed in this case to helping clear and release any karmic energies or traumas that stem from our ancestral forebears.

The first step in the process of healing the family tree is to acquire as much information as possible about the different family members back to the great grandparent generation. In this respect there will be at least fourteen ancestors, including you parents, but you may wish to include aunts and cousins if felt appropriate. There are many online sources now for discovering information about your family. If you do not know anything about your family, perhaps because of adoption, then the healing process can still be worked through. The approach to this healing can be systematic in the sense that you start with your parents and then work backwards through the family tree or it could be based on allowing your intuition linked to your H-S to guide you (Furlong 1997). Additionally these processes can be worked through on your own or with a therapist if felt appropriate. Having someone else to help facilitate can be very helpful.

A typical healing session using this technique would start with an initial discussion followed by a relaxation process that helps the client into a light-trance when the H-S can be accessed. Once the body is fully relaxed a suggestion is made for the client to first access their inner soul essence, which might be perceived as a point or ball of light within the body. Once this place has been accessed then the next step is to connect to the H-S seeing this as wise knowing part of the Self, which is generally recognised as the part of the soul that links directly into the spirit world and has access to various guides and helpers. The H-S part is always fully aware on what is happening within the psyche and within the therapeutic session, yet in respecting the client's free-will only act when requested.

Once the link with the H-S has been established a simple questions can be posed to the H-S for assessing and releasing any traumas. For example, at a very simple level, a request could be made to H-S to reveal whether there is any genetic pattern stemming from the mother (or father) that is present within that creates some form of blockage or influence that affects the client's (or one's own) highest good and to indicate this energy by a colour. If a colour comes to mind it then needs to be cleared under the jurisdiction of the H-S and a colour representing the client's inner soul essence inserted in its place. This process is very simple to follow through and has proved to be very powerful and effective. The client's H-S knows what needs to be done; what energies need to be acknowledged, forgiven, released or integrated. Once complete then the client can be brought back to full waking consciousness. This process can be used for connecting to then clearing and healing all the dynamics and patterns that stem from specific ancestors, such as your great grandmother on your mother's side. In clearing these patterns we do so not only for us but for all family members.

## Conclusions

We all have ancestors and the lives of our ancestors would include a fair level of trauma and conflicting patterns. In some circumstances these might have been dire, filled with anger, fear, hatred and death. Whilst we might be able to shield ourselves from these patterns it is clear that at another level they will continue until healed. The challenge for all healers is to learn to access into their own family trees to heal and balance any traumas that are held therein. The spiritual challenge that we all face is to learn to confront and move through our fears and to learn to love and forgive the unlovable or shameful parts of the self. In more than fifty years as a therapist I would claim that the latter of these two is the most challenging. People find it very difficult to love and forgive themselves. From my own work in ancestral healing the two overwhelming elements that our ancestors seek from us is to be acknowledged and forgiven (Furlong, 1997). We now can be sure that by accessing our Higher-Self we can clear and release these patterns no matter how traumatic they might have been.

## Discussion

One of the challenges for metaphysicians is to find bridges between the physical and the metaphysical sciences. At the moment the world predominantly operates from the stand-point of the known physical sciences and although there are some leading edge researchers prepared to look into the relationship between the physical and spiritual worlds these tend to be in a minority. What is encouraging therefore is when a material science starts to reach a position when possible explanations can be sought from a spiritual understanding. Although there is still a long way to go studies into epigenetics are beginning to raise questions that cannot readily be answered from a materialistic perspective. This perhaps comes to the fore most powerfully in MZ twin studies, which begs the question what is the inherent individuality that would appear to start expressing itself even within the early stages of foetal development. The most plausible explanation is the influence of the incarnating soul. It will perhaps take a moment of epiphany for individual scientists to begin to accept the super-physical and to incorporate this level of awareness into their belief structures. The good news is that this is slowly happening as evidenced by major gatherings, such as the annual Mystics and Scientists conference run by the Scientific and Medical Network in the UK (see SMN https://www.scimednet.org/).

At the other end of life, studies into NDE's are starting to provide mounting evidence for the ability of consciousness to separate from the body that is hard to easily refute if an open mind is kept. This would appear to be some of the best confirmation for the existence of the soul. The problem here is that a mindset that refuses to acknowledge a spiritual component will not easily be persuaded to view life though anything other than the materialistic lens. Perhaps future consciousness studies and the developments within quantum mechanics will break down some of these barriers. The difficulty at the moment is that there is no accepted mechanism for explaining even simple concepts such as telepathy and therefore the easiest stance is to affirm that such experiences cannot occur, expect by pure chance, despite extensive evidence to the contrary. This is the problem with consciousness studies limited to the brain, because, from a neuroscientific perspective, if the soul and brain are indeed two separate entities then how does the soul communicate with and direct its information and intent to the body? It would seem from this viewpoint that there is no discernible pathway of communication. We might liken this to the scientist trying to discover how a television operates working only with the perception that all information must be contained within the TV box, without recognising that this is simply a machine for picking up information from another unseen dimension. Until that bridge is discovered the breaking down of the metaphorical TV box into more and more component parts will go on. If scientists start to hit a dead end in their researches they may then start to look outside of this limited viewpoint and perhaps then we will see some radical breakthroughs.

The evidence that comes forward from researches into soul consciousness such as that carried out by Newton and Zinser give much greater insight into the workings of the psyche and if these systems and models can be shown to be helpful for treating illness and disease a case starts to be built for their acceptance. From my own experience of working as a therapist for more than forty years I can attest for their effectiveness. In whatever way the Higher-Self is perceived, whether it is simply an aspect of the psyche or as an intrinsic part of the soul, the empirical evidence is overwhelming: there is a knowledge and an understanding that we can access within our psyche that can help to resolve many deep seated conditions. In working recently with a client who had been suffering with abuse issues from childhood and had tried all manner of different treatments both orthodox and complimentary over more than thirty years, her connection to her sub-personalities was the start of beginning to clear some of these past blockages. This was to her a revelation. From her perspective is it the only system that has come anywhere close to beginning to solve her healing issues. This type of success can begin to provide a bridge into a growing acceptance of the importance of the metaphysical approach to therapy.

The concept presented by Dr K. McAll that ancestral patterns can influence the psyche is now being accepted by scientists, whereas when his book was written this was regarded as nonsense. Researchers have not yet quite accepted the full gamut of experience that can be passed on to future generations as time has not yet allowed for follow ups to the grandchildren and great grandchildren of some of the study cases. Studies on mice and rats cannot really assess the emotional and psychological dimension of the rodents, although some inherited stress patterns have been observed. My own research into the influence of ancestral patterns supports McAll's thesis and numbers of my clients have had their symptoms alleviated when healing their family tree. The encouraging evidence is that the past is not fixed as original posited by has a fluidity that can be consciously amended and the slate swept clean. It is an encouraging thought that perhaps in future incarnations we will be able to enter into a life where all of our family and personal karma has been cleansed.

## General Conclusions and Summary

Recent studies into epigenetics shows that the way that the patterns within us can be readily adapted and amended. At the moment biological research is focused on manipulating these patterns through forms of medication. However there is also clear evidence that the mind alone has the power to change the manifestation of the patterns as evidenced by the case of the boy with Ichthyosis and the remarkable healing of Anita Moorjani from advanced lymphoma. The power of this process can be further enhanced when access is made to the Soul or Higher-Self part of our being, which has the insights and power to correct and change those aspects that are in need of help. Although it is quite possible to block the patterns of ancestral energy that flow down to us from our family tree, the better approach is to enter into and clear any trauma that is held there, so that future generations might benefit; for when we clear these patterns for ourselves we also clear them for all future generations.

## Bibliography

Appel, Philip. (2003) *The Use of Hypnosis in Physical Medicine and Rehabilitation* Demos Medical Publishing
http://www.ncbi.nlm.nih.gov/books/NBK11206/

Bouchard, Tom. (1994) *Genes, Environment and Personality* Science, New Series, Vol 264, Iss. 5166 (June 17 1994) 1700-1701

Bray, William. (2013) *Quantum Physics, Near Death Experiences, Eternal Consciousness, Religion and the Human Soul* Kindle Edition pub. Createspace

Carey, Nessa. (2013) *The Epigenetic Revolution: How Modern Biology is Rewriting our Understanding of Genetics, Disease and Inheritance* Kindle Edition pub. Icon Books Ltd

Caroll, Robert. (2014) *Near Death Experience (NDE)* SKeptics Online Dictionary see http://www.skepdic.com/nde.html

Chu, James. (2005) *Guidelines for Treating Dissociative Identity Disorder in Adults - 2005* Journal of Trauma & Dissociation, Vol. 6(4) 2005 p.117-118

Eddy, Mary-Baker. (1875) *Science and Health: With Key to the Scriptures* Boston, US

Furlong, David. (1997) *Healing Your Family Patterns: How to access the past to heal the present* Piatkus

Holiday, Robin. (1990) *Mechanisms for the control of gene activity during development.* Biol Rev Camb Philos Soc 65 (4): 431–71.

Kelsey, Denys & Grant, *Joan. (1969) Many Lifetimes* Littlehampton Book Services Ltd

Kübler-Ross, Elizabeth. (2011) YouTube Interview see http://www.youtube.com/watch?v=8uNGhCBOmCg

Mason, Albert. (1952) *Case of Congenital Ichthyosiform Erythrodermia of Brocq treated by Hypnosis* Br Med J 1952;2:422

McAll, Kenneth. (1982) *Healing the Family Tree* Sheldon Press

Moody, Raymond. (1975) *Life After Life: Investigation of a Phenomenon – Survival of Bodily Death* Mockingbird Books

Moorjani, Anita. (2012) *Dying to Be Me: My Journey from Cancer to Near Death to True Healing* Hay House UK Ltd

Motoyama, Hiroshi. (1992) *Karma & reincarnation: The Key to Spiritual Evolution & Enlightenment* Piatkus

Newton, Michael. (1995) *Journey of Souls: Case Studies of Life Between Lives* Llewellyn Publications

Newton, Michael. (2002) *Destiny of Souls: New Case Studies of Life Between Lives* Llewellyn Publications

Newton, Michael. (2004) *Life Between Lives: Hypnotherapy for Spiritual Regression* Llewellyn Publications

Noble, Kim. (2011) *All of Me: My incredible true story of how I learned to live with the many personalities sharing my body* Piatkus

Sabom, Michael. (1998) *Light and Death: One Doctor's Fascinating Account of Near Death Experiences* Zondervan

Sartori, Penny. (2014) *Wisdom of Near Death Experiences: How Understanding of NDE's Can Help Us Live More Fully* Watkins Publishing Ltd

Spector, Timothy. (2012) *Identically Different: Why You Can Change Your Genes* Kindle Edition pub. Weidenfeld & Nicolson

Sykes, Bryan. (2001) *The Seven Daughters of Eve* Bantam Press

Zinser, Tom (2011) *Soul Centred Healing: A Psychologist's Extraordinary Journey into the Realms of Sub-Personalities, Spirits and Past Lives* Union Street Press

# Bibliography and Recommended Reading List

**Foreword**

Hintze, R (2006) *Healing Your Family History*, Hay House

O'Sullivan, N , Graydon, N (2013) *The Ancestral Continuum*, Simon and Schuster

Spector, T. (2012) *Identically Different: Why You Can Change Your Genes* Kindle Edition pub. Weidenfeld & Nicolson

Sykes, B (2001) *The Seven Daughters of Eve*, Bantam Press

Vermont, B & Akey, J (2014) *Resurrecting Surviving Neandertal Lineages from Modern Human Genomes*, Science vol. 343 no 6174, pp 1017-1021

**Introduction**

Motoyama, Hiroshi. (1992) *Karma & reincarnation: The Key to Spiritual Evolution & Enlightenment* Piatkus

McAll, K (1982) *Healing the Family Tree,* Shadow Press

**Chapter 1**

Motoyama, H (1992) *Karma and Reincarnation*, Piatkus

McAll, K (1982) *Healing the Family Tree,* Shadow Press

**Chapter 2**

Moody, R (1978) *Life After Life,* Bantam

Grey, M (1985) *Return from Death,* Arkana

Kübler-Ross, E (1970) *On Death and Dying,* Tavistock

Turman, R. (1994) *The Tibetan Book of the Dead,* Aquarian

Stevenson, I (1974) *Twenty Cases Suggestive of Reincarnation,* University Press, Charlottesville

Kelsey, D & Grant, J (1967) *Many Lifetimes,* Doubleday

Davidson, J (1992) *Natural Creation of Natural Selection,* Element

**Chapter 3**

Anguin, R (1994) *Riding the Dragon,* Element

Arrien, A (1993) *The Four-Fold Way,* HarperCollins

Conrad, J (1998) *The Power of Myth,* Doubleday

Forge, O (1976) *A Pictorial History of the American Indians*: Bonanza Books

Fu-Feng, G & English, J (1989) *Tao Te Ching (Translation),* Vantage Books

Mudrooroo (1994) *Aboriginal Mythology,* Aquarian

Palmer, M, Ramsay, J & Xiaomin, X (1995) *I Ching,* Thorson

Sproul, B (1979) *Primal Myths,* Rider

Stewart, R (1990) *Celtic Gods Celtic Goddesses,* Blandford

Versluis, A (1993) *Native American Traditions,* Element

Waters, F (1963) *The Book of the Hopi,* Ballantine Books

Wilhelm, R (1968) *I Ching: (Translation)* Routledge, Kegan & Paul

Wing, R (1982) *The Illustrated I Ching,* Aquarian

Ywahoo, D (1987) *Voices of Our Ancestors,* Shambala

## Chapter 4

Dossey, L (1993) *Healing Breakthroughs:* Piatkus

Kendler, K.S., et al (2006) A Swedish National Twin Study of Lifetime Major Depression , AMJ Psychiatry, Jan; 163 (1) pp 109-114

Oesterreich, T (1996) *Possession: Demoniacal and Other:* University Books, New York

Silventoinen, K, et al (2003) *Heritability of Adult Body Height: A Comparative Study of Twin Cohorts in Eight Countries,* Twin Research Volume 6 Number 5 pp. 399-408

Woolger, R (1994) *Other Lives, Other Selves:* Aquarian

## Chapter 5

Chopra, D (1989) *Quantum Healing:* Bantam

Sheldrake, R (1989) *The Presence of the Past:* Fontana

Watson, P (1984) *Twins:* Sphere

## Chapter 6

Field, A (1982) *Tracing Your Ancestors,* Treasure Press

McGoldrick, M & Gerson, R (1985) *Genograms in Family Assessment:* Norton and Co

Saul,P (1995) *Tracing Your Ancestors — The A-Z Guide:* Countryside Books

### Chapter 7

Bell, A (1965) *Practical Dowsing:* Bell & Sons

Bradshaw, J (1995) *Family Secrets,* Piatkus

de France, H (1977) *The Elements of Dowsing:* Bell & Sons

Furlong, D (2008) *Develop Your Intuition and Psychic Power:* Atlanta Books

Graves, T (1986) *The Diviner's Handbook:* Aquarian

LeShan, L (1978) *Clairvoyant Reality,* Thorsons

Olsen, D (1990) *Knowing Your Intuitive Mind,* Crystalline Publications

Williamson, T (1993) *Dowsing:* Robert Hale

### Chapter 8

Chambers, C (2006) *End of Life Rituals,* Cherry Tree Books

Wing, R. L (1982) *The Illustrated I Ching:* Aquarian

### Chapters 9 & 10

Angelo, J (1994) *Your Healing Power:* Piatkus

Brennan, B (1988) *Hands of Light:* Bantam

Brennan, B (1993) *Light Emerging:* Bantam

Cade, M & Coxhead, N (1979) *The Awakened Mind:* Wildwood House

Furlong, D (1998) *The Healer Within,* Piatkus

Joy, B (1979) *Joy's Way,* Tarcher

Krieger, D (1979) *Therapeutic Touch,* Prentice Hall

Taylor, A (1987) *I Fly Out With Bright Feathers,* Fontana

Young, A (1981) *Spiritual Healing:* DeVorss

Spindrift Organization *http://www.spindriftresearch.org/*

### Chapter 11

Furlong, D (2003) *Working With Earth Energies,* Piatkus

Linn, D (1995) *Sacred Space,* Rider

Roosbach, S (1986) *Feng Shui,* Rider

Underwood, P (1993) *The Ghost Hunter's Almanac,* Eric Dobby

Walters, D (1988) *Feng Shui,* Pagoda

# Glossary

**Acupuncture:** A system of healing developed in Ancient China over four thousand years ago. It is based on the ability of the acupuncturist to balance a subtle energy known as Ch'i which can be either stimulated or depressed through the insertion of fine needles at specific points of the body. These points are connected through fourteen primary channels (meridians) that are located on the surface of the body and are, in turn, linked to all the internal organs.

**Angel cards:** A set of fifty cards which have single words such as 'Spontaneity', 'Tenderness', 'Enthusiasm' and so on together with a simple drawing of an angel performing an action representing the word. These cards can be obtained from *The Findhorn Foundation, The Park, Forres, 1V36 OTZ, Scotland.*

**Aromatherapy:** A therapy that uses distilled aromatic oils which are absorbed into the body through massage, taken in baths or through direct inhalation.

**Automatic writing:** Written information obtained by putting the mind into an altered state of consciousness. By blocking out conscious thought processes, access is obtained directly to the subconscious mind which can in turn access into the 'collective unconscious'.

**Aura:** The composite energy fields that surround all life forms.

**Bach remedies:** Discovered by Dr Bach in the 1930s this therapeutic system uses flower essences to improve emotional states which Bach saw as one of the primary causes of disease. Information on these remedies can be obtained from *The Bach Centre, Mount Vernon, Sotwell, Wallingford, Oxon OX10 OPZ, tel: 01491 834678.*

**Beast of Albion cards:** Produced by Miranda Grey, this set of cards depicts thirty-nine different animals associated with Britain in a natural or mythological way. Each animal portrays specific psychological types or states of mind and can therefore be used as a system of inner development. The set can be acquired through HarperCollins publishers.

**Carl Jung:** Swiss psychiatrist who founded the analytical psychology movement. He lived from 1875 to 1961.

**Chakras:** Vortices of energy generally along the front of the body that connect the spiritual realm to the physical. There are traditionally said to be seven main chakras.

**Cellular memory:** The ability of the cells of the body to hold memories or information relevant to the life of the individual. It is now known that these memories can be carried over in transplant operations where the receiver can pick up information about the donor of the organ, even taking on some of their previous psychological traits.

**Ch'i:** Derived from Ancient Chinese system of medicine, Ch'i is said to be a subtle energy of the cosmos that provides form and sustenance to the manifest world. This energy can be manipulated to an extent by conscious thought.

**Christian Science healing:** Developed by Mary Baker Eddy in the USA following a miraculous recovery from a skating accident. It is based on the recognition of a perfected spiritual essence that is claimed to be within all human beings. Disease is said to be a failure to recognise this inner perfection that knows no imbalance or illness. It could be summed up in the following precept. 'God is perfect, we are all a reflection of God, we only need to affirm that perfection to be whole and well.' Christian Science was formalized into a religion in 1875.

**Chromosomes:** Threadlike, microscopic structures found in the nuclei of cells. They are formed of DNA and protein and comprise chains of genes.

**Crystal therapy:** Crystals are claimed to be able to focus and amplify healing energy which is then directed to areas of imbalance within the patient. By placing the right stone into the energy field of the body, beneficial changes can be generated.

**Disease:** Disharmony or conflict at any level between or within the different elements that link the physical to spiritual body. This principle applies to all life forms, but in human beings is seen broadly as relating to the physical, emotional, mental and spiritual aspects of our make-up.

**Distant healing:** The projection of healing energy (Ch'i) to someone or something not present with the healer.

**DNA:** Deoxyribonucleic acid; the basic life molecule that contains the genetic code that is found within each cell of a living organism.

**Dowsing:** A method of obtaining information, using either a pendulum, divining rod or other implement which magnify the subtle sensations of the physical body.

**Dualism:** The philosophical notion of two distinct principles existing in all things. Similar to the concepts of yin/yang but generally carrying an idea that one is opposed to the other like good or bad or light or dark. Within human beings this is taken to mean that the mind or soul and the physical body are two separate entities often at conflict with each other.

**Ego mind:** The aspect of the self, aware of its individuality, that has a consciousness of and reflects the different elements of the physical world. Therefore it tends to respond more readily to the needs and appetites of the physical and emotional self as opposed to the Spiritual-Self.

**Energy:** A force that has an ability or capacity to produce an effect on whatever it is directed towards.

**Exorcism:** The process of removing a 'spirit' presence from a space, such as a house, or from a person.

**Family therapy:** Considers the family both past and present as a single unit in which the individual members are facts of the whole. The method seeks to: 1) engage the whole family in the therapeutic process; 2) unblock the system; 3) clarify family patterns; and 4) to reframe and detoxify family issues'. (McGoldrick and Gerson, see p.99).

**Genes:** DNA molecules that shape inherited characteristics.

**Ghost:** The manifestation of an 'earth' bound spirit.

**Guides:** Spirit beings who assist incarnate individuals.

**Guided imagery:** This is the use of a sequence of imaged exercises that induces different psychological or emotional states. Images, such as those that appear in dreams, act as keys to the deepest layers of consciousness.

**Healer:** One who consciously projects out healing energy or attempts to bring harmony and balance to another.

**Healing:** This is the process of adjustment that seeks wholeness or balance. This can either be experienced within the self or projected out towards another.

**Higher-Self:** The aspect of the Spiritual-Self that is directly in touch with the spiritual realm as opposed to the soul which is the aspect of the Spiritual-Self that connects through to the mind and body.

**Homeopathy:** Based on the ancient concepts that 'like treats like,' it was first systematized by Samuel Hahnemann in 1796. It involves the dilution to minute quantities of a wide variety of substances that are known to produce specific symptoms when taken in their undiluted form. The homeopath tries to match the correct homeopathic remedy with the symptoms of the patient. Hahnemann also believed that certain inherited illness tendencies known as miasms could be passed on to the future generations. If suppressed or not treated correctly these could erupt in a more violent form either within the patient or his or her offspring.

**Hypnotism:** A process of trance induction that by-passes some aspects of the 'Ego mind' to gain access to the deeper layers of the self.

**I Ching:** Literally the 'Book of Changes', that stems from Ancient China. It formed a divinatory oracle that was used to gain insights into the prevailing spiritual forces in operation around the question asked, so helping the querent make the right decision.

**Jing:** Ancestral energy expressed both through sexual release and the genetic coding stemming from Taoist and Ancient Chinese beliefs.

**Karma:** The Hindu and Buddhist belief based on the law of cause and effect.

**Law of polarities:** See yin/yang.

**Mantra:** A word that is repeated either audibly or inwardly as part of meditation discipline.

**Medicine cards:** A set of cards based on Native American animal symbols, such as the bear, buffalo and coyote. Like other similar systems (see Beast of Albion) each animal is attributed certain human characteristics. Selecting a card or cards highlights those aspects as relevant for the moment they are drawn.

**Meditation:** A generic word covering a wide range of different mental methods of connecting to the inner source of our being.

**Mind:** An aspect of the self that is the seat of conscious and subconscious awareness. It bridges between the Spiritual-Self and the emotions.

**Morphic Resonance**: A concept postulated by biologist Rupert Sheldrake whereby the memories or habits of nature are communicated within species and across generations. This information is held within a 'morphogenic field' which surrounds and links together all living things.

**Mudras:** A system of inner development based upon holding the hands in set positions. These poses create a resonant energy that links together different aspects of the self.

**Nature/nurture debate:** A long standing debate that has engaged many scientific minds and studies in the evaluation of human personality. In simple terms it has tried to determine how much of our characteristics are derived from our upbringing (nurture) as opposed to our genetic inheritance (nature). The implications of the resolution of this debate are profound for it can and has shaped political systems sometimes, as in the case of Nazism, with disastrous results.

**Near death experience (NDE)**: A widely based experience which generally occurs when the physical body seems to die, but can sometimes happen spontaneously. In the experience, part of the consciousness appears to detach itself from the body and is aware of what is taking place from a perspective separate from the body. Sometimes these individuals will then feel that they are travelling through a tunnel into another dimension where they often report meeting others who they know have already died.

**Neuro-linguistic programming (NLP):** The art and science of personal excellence founded by John Grinder and Richard Bandler. Based upon a study of three famous therapists it was perceived they used similar underlying patterns in resolving problems. NLP tries to reframe the way that we think about our reality to bring about change.

**Noble middle path:** A tenet of Buddhism that seeks a balance between extremes.

**Numerology:** A system of analysis of underlying principles by reducing everything to number. Of ancient origin it forms part of Hebrew tradition, where it is known as gematria, as well as being an aspect of Pythagorean teaching. Each letter of the alphabet is ascribed a number and so individual names or words can be reduced to a number by adding up the individual parts. These numbers are then interpreted by the exponent.

**Olympus cards:** Devised by Murry Hope these cards are based on Greek mythological characters. They can be obtained from HarperCollins publishers.

**Osteopathy:** A system of treatment based on the manipulation of the joints of the body.

**Past-life therapy:** A system of healing that seeks to bring relief to behavioural patterns that stem from a past-life experience.

**Personality types:** A method of categorizing human characteristics under a number of set headings. At its simplest level it classes individuals as either introverted or extroverted.

**Placebo effect:** The recognition that the belief of the subject will in itself aid a cure. Clinical double-blind trials using sugar-based pills with no other additives have shown that marked improvements occur in about 30 per cent of patients if there is a belief in the efficacy of the substance being administered. This effect is now taken into account in all clinical trials.

**Psi healing:** Another name for spiritual healing. The word 'psi' is now used in scientific paranormal studies as opposed to the word 'psychic' because of the latter's biased associations.

**Psyche:** From Greek, meaning `breath' and is taken to refer to the human soul or inner motivating life force.

**Psychic faculty:** An innate human skill that allows us to communicate with and experience different levels of perception outside of time or space.

**Psychic diagnosis:** A way of using the psychic faculty to gain insights and information not apparent from the five physical senses.

**Psycho-kinetic:** The ability of the mind to influence physical objects, apparatus or machinery causing them to move or change in ways outside of the known laws of physics.

**Radionics:** A system of vibrational treatment first developed by Albert Abrams in the USA in the early part of the twentieth century. Originally based on the idea that each substance or disease state produced a radiating electromagnetic energy at a consistent specific set frequency that could be readily measured. Abrams used this system to diagnose conditions within his patients. In modern times the concept has been expanded to consider that these emanations originate from an etheric or non-physical level. To effect treatment the radionic practitioner broadcasts back the correcting frequencies to produce the required changes.

**Reflexology:** A system of treatment based on the massage of the feet. Reflexologists consider that different areas of the feet relate to the different organs of the body. By gentle massage to tender spots healing energy can be channelled to imbalanced areas.

**Regression:** An induced mental state either by another or through oneself to access below the normal layers of the conscious mind.

**Reiki healing:** A system of healing similar to spiritual or psi healing. It was developed in the nineteenth century by Mikao Usui a Japanese Christian theologian, who claimed to have rediscovered ancient Tibetan healing practices and reinterpreted them in the light of the healing methods of Jesus.

**Reincarnation:** The belief that each soul lives a number of separate and distinct lives. Resonance: A concept that explains how energy is transferred between things or people on a non-physical level. Based on the notion that when two objects are pitched musically at the same frequency energy is exchanged between them.

**Runes:** An ancient Norse and Teutonic magical alphabet used for divination and casting spells.

**Shaman**: A word that has recently taken on a wide meaning. Originally referred to the 'magician spirit healers' of Finland and Central Asia, it is now applied widely to all individuals who espouse similar beliefs. One of the main magical symbols of the shaman is the drum which is used to summon up spiritual energy or spirit beings.

**Shen:** The 'spirit' in Taoist and Ancient Chinese belief.

**Shiatsu:** A system of healing derived from Japan that uses finger pressure and massage to the acupuncture meridians of the body.

**Shinto:** The native religion of Japan that sees spiritual life in all things. Particularly venerated are the ancestral spirits of the clan or family.

**Soul:** The aspect of the spirit that directly links into the body.

**Spirit:** The external divine part of the Self that contains the sum total of all individual experiences, whether from this life or previous lives.

**Spiritual healing:** The concept that healing energy can be channelled through the mind of an individual and directed towards another to assist the self-healing mechanisms of the body. The main difference between many similar systems of healing is where each sees the source of this healing energy. Religious based systems place this with God, whilst others would see it as a universal energy. (See Reiki healing, Psi healing, Christian Science healing).

**Spiritual-Self:** Another way of describing the spirit *(see above).*

**Tarot:** A divinatory system based on seventy-eight cards that are divided into a Major Arcana of twenty-two cards and Minor Arcana of fifty-six cards.

**Tao:** 'The Way'; understood in Ancient Chinese and Taoist belief to mean the 'way of right action'.

**Telepathy:** The ability of the mind to communicate directly with another mind across space and time.

**Yin/Yang:** The concept developed in Ancient China that perceived everything within the formative and manifest world being based upon the interplay of two forces, that are both opposite and complementary at the same time. Yang is the outgoing principle, whilst yin is receptive.

**Yoga:** The word is derived from the Sanskrit and means 'union with the Spiritual-Self', with different body postures to attain higher states of consciousness.

# Useful Addresses

**David Furlong** Training Courses:
> Myrtles, Como Road, Malvern, Worcs WR14 2TH. Tel: 0777-978-9047
> Websites: www.atlanta-association.com and www.spiritrelease.org
> Email: atlanta@dial.pipex.com

**British Organisations Providing Training Courses in Healing:**

*The College of Healing,* PO Box 342, Malvern, Worcs WR14 9GU. Tel:
> 01684 578963

Website: www.collegeofhealing.org Email: info@CollegeofHealing.org

*The Healing Trust,* 21 York Road, Northampton, NN1 5QG. Tel: 01604
> 603247

*British Alliance of Healing Associations*
> www.britishalliancehealingassociations.com/

*The White Eagle Lodge,* Brewell Lane, Rake, Liss, Hants. Tel: 01730 893300

*Spiritualist Association of Great Britain,* 33 Belgrave Square, London
> W1. Tel: 0171-235 3351

*Sufi Healing Order of Great Britain,* www.sufihealingorderuk.org/

**General**

*American Society of Genealogists,* 1228 Eye Street NW, Washington DC
> 20005

*Australian Genealogical Society,* 120 Kent Street, Sydney, NSW

*Births, Deaths and Marriages Office ( Eire ),* 8-11 Lombard Street,
> Dublin 2, Eire

*Federation of Family History Societies,* 96 Beaumont Street,
> Milehouse, Plymouth PL2 3AQ

*Genealogical Society of Latter Day Saints (IGI),* 64-68 Exhibition Road,
> London SW7

*Genealogical Society of Utah,* The Church of Latter Day Saints, Family
> History Library, 35 Northwest Temple, Salt Lake City, Utah
> 84150, USA

*Genealogical Society of South Africa,* PO Box 4839, Cape Town 8000

*General Register Office,* St Catherine's House, 10 Kingsway, London
> WC2B 6JB

*General Register Office (Scotland),* New Register House, Edinburgh EH1 3YT

*General Register Office ( Northern Ireland),* 49-55 Chichester Street, Belfast BT1 4HL

*Public Records Office,* Ruskin Avenue, Kew, Richmond, SY TW9 4DU

*Society of Genealogists,* 14 Charterhouse Buildings, London EC1

**Websites**

*Ancestry.com* http://home.ancestry.co.uk/

*Find My Past* http://www.findmypast.co.uk/

*Genes Reunited* http://www.genesreunited.co.uk/home/index

*Genuki* http://www.genuki.org.uk/


All correspondence regarding training courses run by David Furlong should be sent address given at the top.

**Bank Ancestral Chart**

A blank ancestral chart (see p.75) can be downloaded from the following link:

http://www.kch42.dial.pipex.com/pdf/ancestorchart1.pdf

# Index